GASTROINTESTINAL STROMAL TUMOR

Edited by **Raimundas Lunevicius**

Gastrointestinal Stromal Tumor
Edited by Raimundas Lunevicius

Published by InTech
Janeza Trdine 9, 51000 Rijeka, Croatia

Publishing Process Manager Bojan Rafaj

Technical Editor Teodora Smiljanic

Cover Designer InTech Design Team

Additional hard copies can be obtained from orders@intechopen.com

Gastrointestinal Stromal Tumor, Edited by Raimundas Lunevicius
p. cm.
ISBN 978-953-51-0580-0

For EU product safety concerns:
IN TECH d.o.o., Prolaz Marije Krucifikse Kozulić 3, 51000 Rijeka, Croatia,
info@intechopen.com or visit our website at intechopen.com.

Meet the editor

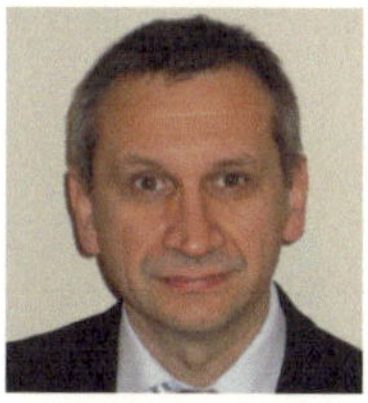

Dr Raimundas Lunevicius, MD, PhD, Dr Sc, FRCS, qualified at Vilnius University, Lithuania, in 1986. He trained in general surgery at acute care hospitals in Lithuania (1986-1996), Kristianstad General Hospital, (1996, Sweden), and Nagoya University Hospital (1998-2000, Japan). In 1996 he became a senior general surgeon (a consultant post) at Vilnius University Emergency Hospital. In 2004 he became an acting / full professor of general surgery. He completed Monbushou (cancer surgery, 1998–2000, Japan) and Fulbright – Humphrey (trauma systems, 2008–2009, Johns Hopkins University, US) Fellowship Programmes. From 2010 he works for the King's College NHS Foundation Trust, and King's College, University of London. His clinical interest include general, gastrointestinal, emergency & trauma surgery, and his research interests are now focused around acute care surgery and surgery links to global health, Africa. Educator, trainer, supervisor, editor, reviewer, adviser, auditor, organizer, researcher. Author or co-author of more than 130 publications and five books.

Contents

Preface

One year ago I was kindly asked by Ms Ana Pantar and Mr Bojan Rafaj, editorial consultants at *InTech* (www.intechweb.org), leading *Open Access* publisher of scientific books and journals in the science, technology, and medicine fields; to edit the book that would provide comprehensive knowledge on a group of malignant mesenchymal tumours named *gastrointestinal stromal tumours (GISTs)*. I was also asked to write the preface for this book, to which I am delighted to do for both parts. The invitation itself brought up a few questions. What should the style and structure of the book be? Should it be in a form of a textbook or handbook, whereby the titles of chapters reflect a fundamental structure and the content of the educational book (historical overview, epidemiology, genetics, pathology, classifications, clinical presentation, diagnosis, etc.) or should it be a collection of selected comprehensive review articles, reports of original studies, and case presentations, contributed by clinical oncologists, surgeons, pathologists, and researchers from various institutions of Europe, Asia, and the US?

The power of reality was stronger than the power of imagination. We ended up with the kind of book which can be characterized as a collection of review papers mainly on diagnostics and management of GISTs, and a few golden pieces of original research. In this context I think that the fact that 31 authors of the papers, work in different countries and institutions, thus amplified value of their shared reviews, opinions, and unique clinical and pathological experience. A reader of the book, therefore, will be able to find essential knowledge and key facts about gastrointestinal stromal tumours' epidemiology, genetics, molecular biology, etiology, mechanisms of tumor development, pathology, diagnostics, classifications, surgical and conservative management, and prognosis as the book reflects a theory and practise on GISTs. That would mean that the aim of this project for me is – to help the reader to obtain an objective and comprehensive general picture of GISTs, as well as to present a useful and educational reference for physicians and surgeons, residents and medical students – to be achieved. One should be bear in mind before opening the first page of this book, that this special issue dedicated to GISTs lays no claim of encompassing the whole of the GIST problem *per se* in all its multidisciplinary fundamental complexity.

The sequence of the chapters has been chosen in order to highlight areas of current practise, change in management, variability of features of GISTs, and original research. The review *"GISTs: from the history to the tailored therapy"* provided by Roberta

Zappacosta and co-workers (Italy) demonstrates how the GIST, went from being poorly defined, to a treatment-resistant neoplasia which became a well recognised, well understood and effectively treated neoplasia. The second paper *"Treatment Options for Gastrointestinal Stromal Tumors"* written by Kai-Hsi Hsu (Taiwan, Republic of China) was dedicated to the management of GIST with respect to tumour location and disease stage. It emphasises a multidisciplinary team approach in managing patients with GIST. The author expresses a reasonable assumption that future treatment of GIST may move towards individualised targeted therapy in combination with surgery in order to optimise clinical outcomes. The *"Molecularly targeted therapy: imatinib and beyond"* (Andrew Poklepovic and Prithviraj Bose, USA) was focused on the molecular biology of gastrointestinal stromal tumours with emphasis on therapy; targeting the primary activating mutations in the KIT proto-oncogene. The studies that have led to the approval of current adjuvant and neo-adjuvant therapy were effectively reviewed in this paper. The significance of basic research towards a deeper understanding of the primary and secondary mutations of proto-oncogenes is timely pointed out. António M. Gouveia and José Manuel Lopes (Portugal) discuss different aspects of surgical treatment of GISTs. They emphasise that complete surgical resection without lymph node dissection is considered to be a standard treatment for primary localised non-metastatic gastrointestinal stromal tumours, and nowadays, is the only potential curative current treatment for patients. The overview *"The role of the surgeon in multidisciplinary approach to gastrointestinal stromal tumours"* (written by Selim Sözen and co-workers, Turkey) draws limits and shows significance of surgical management of gastrointestinal stromal tumours. Aiwen Wu (PR China) explores the most important aspects of GIST in the anorectum. Mainly, this report includes diagnosis, differential diagnosis, and treatment of anorectal GIST. An interesting and uncommon case of extragastrointestinal stromal tumour located in the rectovaginal septum was described by Josefa Marcos Sanmartín and co-workers (Spain). This excellent case report with literature review demonstrates necessity and the importance of considering 'extragastrointestinal stromal tumours' in the differential diagnosis of mesenchymal neoplasms in the vulvovaginal-rectovaginal septum. The paper written by Ardeleanu Carmen Maria and Enache Simona (Romania) explores variability of the histopathological, immunohistochemical and molecular features of gastrointestinal stromal tumours. Again, it shows that the idea to profile an individual patient's GIST mutations is of paramount importance for targeted therapy. Keishiro Aoyagi, Kikuo Kouhuji, and Kazuo Shirouzu (Japan) presented results of original clinicopathological and immunohistochemical study. They assessed the reliabilities of the Ki-67 labeling index, the expression of c-kit, p53, and bcl-2, and the apoptotic count for predicting potential malignancy of gastrointestinal stromal tumour. Finally, a meta-analysis aimed to derive a more precise estimation of the relationship between p53 and biologic behaviour of gastrointestinal stromal tumour was performed by Zong Liang, and Chen Ping. Evidence from 19 studies including 1163 patients, was gained and discussed in a highly conclusive manner. In short, despite the fact that there have been some manuscripts on GISTs in the past; I am pleased to see this book on gastrointestinal stromal tumours. I salute the authors for their professional dedication and outstanding work in summarizing their clinical and research practices with established and upcoming theories on GISTs, as this always helps to implement better management procedures to a given standard.

Raimundas Lunevicius MD, PhD, Dr Sc, FRCS
[1]King's College Hospital NHS Foundation Trust, London,
[2]Professor of General Surgery, Vilnius University,
[1]United Kingdom
[2]Lithuania

1

GISTs: From the History to the Tailored Therapy

Roberta Zappacosta, Barbara Zappacosta, Serena Capanna,
Chiara D'Angelo, Daniela Gatta and Sandra Rosini
Oncology and Experimental Medicine Department, Cytopathology Unit,
G. d'Annunzio University of Chieti-Pescara
Italy

1. Introduction

Gastrointestinal stromal tumours (GISTs) represent the most common non-epithelial mesenchymal tumours of the gastrointestinal tract. The role of the pathologist in the differential diagnosis of GISTs, as well as the correct understanding of these neoplasia by detailed clinicopathologic, biological and genetic studies, are becoming increasingly important in optimizing the management of these tumours and to develop new therapies for the treatment of advanced diseases.

2. Historical overview

At the beginning there were more misunderstandings about GIST. On the basis of light microscopic descriptions and until 1960, Gastrointestinal Stromal Tumors (GISTs) were though to be neoplasms of smooth muscle origin; so they were classified as leiomyoma, leyomiosarcoma or leyomioblastoma, in one word STUMP (Smooth-muscle Tumors of Undetermined malignant Potential). In the early 1970s, electron microscopic studies revealed inconsistent evidence of smooth muscle differentiation. During '80s, this data was supported by the application of immunohistochemical studies, which showed that the expression of muscle markers (such as actins and desmins) was far more variable than those observed in smooth muscle tumors arising from the myometrium. Immunohistochemistry also demonstrated the existence of a subset of stromal neoplasia having neural crest immunophenotype (S100- and neuron-specific enolase - NSE-positivity) which has not been found in other smooth muscle neoplasms. These findings switched on a long-standing debate about the real origin and nature of mesenchymal tumors arising within the gut wall. In 1983, Mazur and Clark postulated the derivation of these "stromal tumors" from mesenchymal stem element, considered to be the progenitor of both spindle and epithelioid cells, and showing CD34 positivity. In 90s, it began to refer to "GISTs" to collectively designate a group of mesenchymal tumours with miogenic or neurogenic differentiation, arising from gastrointestinal tract, separate from stromal tumors taking place of other sites (e.g. uterus). The observation of both smooth muscle characteristics and neural features in GISTs, led to the conclusion that these tumour would be related to a little population of spindle cells placed in the gut wall. So, in 1998 Kindblom et al, definitively defined the origin of GISTs from a pluripotential stem cell, programmed to differentiate into either

Intestitial Cajal Cell (ICC) and smooth muscle cells. They represent ICCs as a network of cellular elements, intercalated between nerve fibres and muscle cells, involved in the generation of gut contraction (Figure 1).

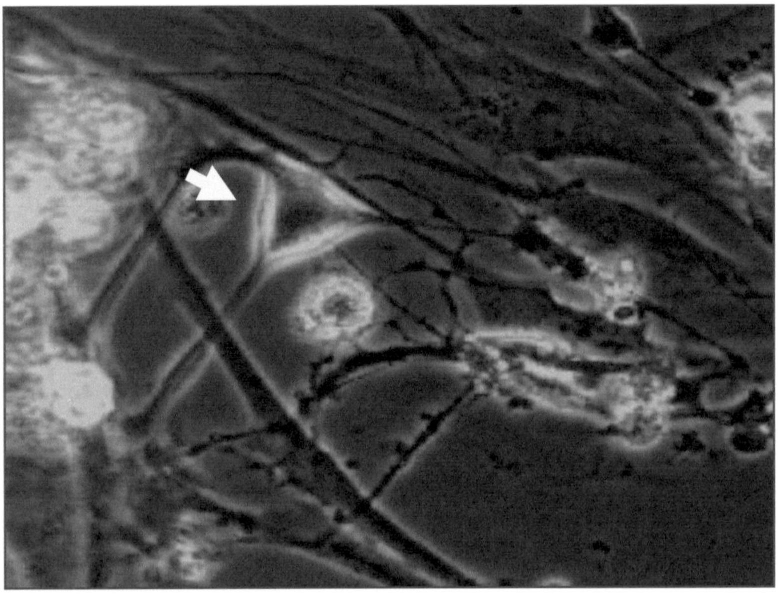

Fig. 1. Cajal cell (arrow) within gastrointestinal wall

Successive studies performed on ICCs demonstrated their growth depending on stem cell factor signalling through KIT tyrosine kinase (CD117) (Isozaki et al., 1995). In 1998, publications by Hirota et al., and Kindblom et al., announced to scientific community the expression of CD117 on GISTs (Kingblom et al., 1998; Miettinen et al., 2005).
Starting from this point, Ogasawara et al. assigned to *c-kit* mutation of ICC an early causal role in GIST tumorigenesis and Agaimy et al. defined GIST as the grossly identifiable counterpart of sporadic ICC hyperplasia.
In subsequent years and to these days, all the previous observations led to the correct classification of GISTs (CD117-positive) as a separate entity from smooth muscle neoplasia (CD117-negative) and to the development of a target-therapy for this disease.

3. c-kit gene, KIT receptor and kit mutations

The c-kit gene is the cellular homologue of the oncogene v-kit of HZ4 feline sarcoma virus, encoding a type III receptor protein-tyrosine kinase (KIT). The type III class of receptors also includes the plateled-derivated growth factor receptors, α and β-chain (PDGFRα, PDGFRβ), the macrophage colony-stimulating factor (M-CSF) receptor and the FI cytokine receptor (Flt3). All protein-tyrosine kinase receptors share the same topology: an extracellular ligand-binding domain, made up five immunoglobulin-like repeats, a single transmembrane sequence, a juxtamembrane domain, that is considered to be significant for regulation of KIT dimerization and in the inhibition of kinase activity, and a cytoplasmic kinase domain (Figure 2). The structure and amino-acid sequence of KIT is well preserved in humans, mices and rats.

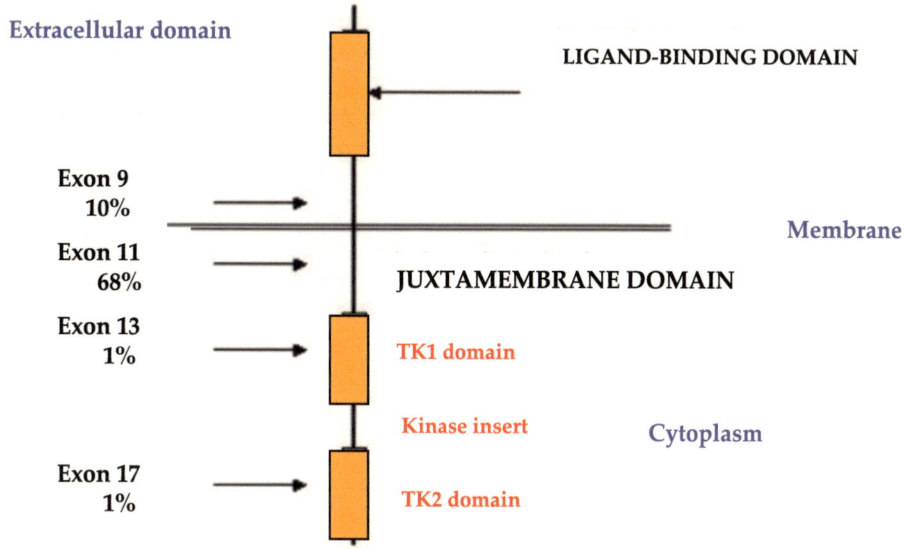

Fig. 2. KIT receptor structure and distribution of KIT mutations

The ligand for KIT is named Stem Cell Factor (SCF); it binds to the second and third immunoglobulin domains, playing the fourth domain a role in receptor dimerization (Zhang et al., 2000). Two molecules of wild-type KIT form a dimer by binding two molecules of SCF; dimerization leads to autophosphorylation of KIT on tyrosine kinase domain and to activation of protein kinase activity through several signal transduction systems, such as phosphatidylinositol 3-kinase (PI3K)/Akt pathway, Ras/mitogen activated protein kinase (MAPK) pathway and jak/STAT pathway (Huizinga et al., 1995; Ullrich et al., 1990). The activation of PI3K/Akt pathway may explain in part how activating mutations of KIT participate in neoplastic transformation.

By the induction of cell proliferation and differentiation, KIT is important in erythropoiesis, lymphopoiesis, mast cell development and functions, megakaryocytopoiesis, gametogenesis and melanogenesis (Rönnstrand, 2004).

In the absence of SCF, KIT exists in a monomeric dormant state. The mechanism for the activation of dormant KIT involves binding of the appropriate ligand to the extracellular domain of two receptor monomers; this connection produces a receptor dimer. SCF also exists as a non-covalent dimer, which binds to two KIT monomers, thereby promoting KIT dimer formation (Zhang et al., 2000).

In 1988, c-kit gene was founded at the W locus of mouse chromosome 5. The W locus of mice encodes KIT. Many types of loss-of-function mutants have been reported at the W locus. The W mutant allele is a point mutation at the tyrosine kinase (TK) domain, resulting in a dramatic decreasing of TK activity. Heterozygotic W-wild/W-mutated mices show five abnormalities due to the loss of KIT function: 1) anemia, due to hypoproduction of erytrocytes; 2) white coat colour, due to the lack of melanocytes; 3) sterility, due to the depletion of germ cells; 4) depletion of mast cells; 5) depletion of ICCs.

Molecular analyses of the c-kit gene in *W* mutants facilitated the understanding of the in vivo function of KIT (Hayashi et al., 1991). In 1992, Maeda et al., analyzing c-kit expression in phenotipically normal mouse tissues, demonstrated c-kit expression in healthy mouse.

Particularly, they showed the presence of KIT-positive cells in GI muscular layers, especially in the myenteric plexus layer. Distribution of KIT-positive cells seemed similar to that of ICC cells.
Subsequently, many types of loss-of-function mutant mice have reported at the W locus. Myenteric plexus ICCs fail to develop in mice which are deficient in expression of the KIT tyrosine kinase receptor or in its ligand SCF, indicating that the KIT-SCF axis is essential for the development of these cells. *W* mutant mice, who had deficiency of KIT-positive cells, also had disturbed GI movements, including bile reflux to stomach. These results unequivocally demonstrated that ICC are KIT-positive and that pacemaker of GI movement is KIT-dependent (Maeda H et al., 1992). Actually, it is well known that loss-of-function mutations of KIT also result in mast cells depletion.
In >80% of GISTs, mutation in the c-kit gene leads to KIT constitutive activation (gain-of-function mutation). Activating KIT mutations occur in the extracellular, in the juxtamembrane and in the proximal and distal protein kinase domains (Table 1), and more often consist in single oligonucleotide substitution in exon 11. The penetrance appears to be high.
Since KIT plays an essential role in development of melanocytes and mast cells, most individuals with exon 11 mutations may also develop mast cell disease, as well as hyperpigmentation of perineal, perioral and digital skin area. This fact does not occur for patients with a KIT exon 13 or 17 mutations, suggesting that there are differences in signalling requirements for mast cells neoplasia as compared with GISTs.

Tumor type	Location of mutation in KIT
GIST	Extracellular domain
Mast cell leukemia	JM segment
Germ-cell tumor	JM segment
Mastocytosis	JM segment
GIST	Proximal kinase domain
Germ-cell tumor, GIST, mastocytosis	Activation loop
Germ-cell tumor, GIST	Activation loop
Seminoma	Activation loop
T-cell lymphomas	Activation loop

Table 1. Oncogenic gain-of-function KIT mutations, in human

The most common mutations in KIT affect the juxtamembrane domain encoding exon 11. Two-third of GISTs harbour an inframe deletion, insertion, substitution or combination of this exon (Figure 1), while approximately 10% of these neoplasia have a mutation in an extracellular domain encoded by exon 9. Rarely, mutations occur in the kinase I (exon 13) and kinase II (exon 17) domains.
In human mast cell leukemia cell line HMC-1, KIT is constitutively phosphorylated in kinase domain, activated and then associated with PI3K without the addition of SCF. c-kit gene of HMC-1 cells is composed of normal-wild-type allele and of mutant allele having point mutations which result in the substitution of Val-560 to Gly in juxtamembrane domain, and Asp-816 to Val in tyrosine kinase domain.
In a transfected cells model, KIT with either mutations is phosphorylated on tyrosine and activates without the addition of SCF. The mechanisms of constitutive activation are different in the cases of Val to Gly and Asp to Val. A substantial fraction of phosphorylated

KIT with Val to Gly mutation dimerizes, whereas phosphorylated KIT with Asp to Val mutation does not (Feritsu et al., 1993).

In general, tumors are heterozygous for a given mutation, but loss of the remaining wild-type KIT allele occurs in about 8-15% of tumors; in these cases, there would be a strict association with a wrong prognosis (Corless & Heinrich, 2008). In a subset of GISTs which are wild-type, a high proportion have mutations in either exon 12 or 18 of the plateled-derived growth factor alpha (PDGFα) gene. PDGFα substitution in exon 18 is only found in GISTs arising in the stomach, mesentery and omentum.

The importance of KIT mutation in GISTs development is sustained by numerous evidences. First, when expressed in transfected cell lines, mutant form of KIT show constitutive kinase activity in the absence of SCF (Hirota et al., 1998). Second, mutant KIT is oncogenic (Hirota et al., 1998). Third, phosphorylated KIT is detectable in GIST. Fourth, patients with hereditary mutations are at high risk for the development of multiple GISTs. Fifth, mice engineered to express mutant KIT shows ICC cell hyperplasia and develops stromal tumors resembling human GISTs (Rubin et al., 2005).

4. Interstitial cells of Cajal (ICC) and GISTs

ICCs were firstly described by Santiago Ramon y Cajal in 1983, as special cells distinct from ordinal neurons, forming a network in the GI wall of the Guinea pigs (Cajal, 1983). ICC act as the "pacemaker" cell of the gut and serve as intermediaries between the GI autonomic nervous system and smooth cells, to regulate GI motility and coordinate peristalsis. Although location and density of ICCs vary in different portion of GI tract, the largest density of these cells occurs around the myenteric plexus, with extension between intramural neurons and smooth muscular cells of the circular and longitudinal layers of the muscolaris propria.

ICCs are classified into several subtypes by anatomical localization; moreover, a subset of ICCs are known to mediate neural transmission. In this context, ICCs are considered to play different roles. Cajal et al., estimated that ICCs were primitive neurons. Actually it's well known that ICCs would derive from a common precursor that yields ICC and smooth muscle cells, but not neurons (Torihashi et al., 1997).

As previously described, KIT was reported to be expressed by these cells; in fact, ICC requires the SCF-KIT system for its development. Loss-of-function mutation of KIT results in depletion of ICCs. Conversely, gain-of-function mutation might induce ICCs neoplasms. Normal ICCs as well as ICCs neoplasia express CD117. Since leiomyomas and schwannomas did not express KIT, but most tumors designated as GISTs did express it, it has been postulate the origin of GISTs from ICCs.

Although more than 90% of GISTs harbour a specific *c-kit* gene mutation, and approximately 85% of GISTs have mutations in either KIT or PDGFα receptors, recent molecular studies defined a subset of gastrointestinal stromal tumors which are clearly KIT- and PDGFRα-negative (*kit* wild type [*kit*-WT] (Corless et al., 2002).

About 12% of the stromal gastrointestinal tumors lack a KIT mutation. Heinrich et al., investigating the cause of GISTs without KIT mutation and using Western blotting analysis based on a cocktail of antibodies to epitopes pooled by a broad range of tyrosine kinases receptors, revealed a gain-of-function mutations of PDGFα receptor in about one-third of GISTs (Heinrich et al., 2003). Mutated PDGFα receptor activates not only itself, but also wild-type KIT. Since the signal transduction pathway of PDGFα receptor is similar to that of

KIT, gain-of-function mutation of PDGFα receptor by itself may cause transformation of ICCs.
When compared with kit-positive GISTs, kit-WT tumors are more likely to arise in the omentum/peritoneal surface and stomach whereas GISTs kit-positive occurred predominantly in the small bowel. The presence of KIT mutation in GISTs has been correlated with survival of patients. Survival seems better in patients without KIT mutation than in patients without KIT mutation (Taniguchi et al., 1999). Among mutant GISTs, comparative studies indicated different pharmacological responsiveness to the kinase inhibitor *imantinib.*
It is now widely accepted that mutations of other genes are also necessary for GIST to emerge from a background of ICC hyperplasia. Particularly, some tumor suppressor genes which are closely correlated with tumorigenesis, have been found to harbour abnormalities in GISTs. Recently, functional inactivation of $p16^{INK4a}$ gene transcript on 9p21 locus, via mutation, deletion, or promoter hypermethylation, causing loss or down-regulation of the corresponding protein, has been identified as an independent unfavourable prognostic factor in GISTs (Ricci et al., 2004; Sabah et al., 2004; Schneider et al., 2003; Scheneider-Stock et al., 2005).
$p16^{INK4a}$ is one of the two alternative transcripts of the cyclin-dependent kinase inhibitor 2A (CDKN2A) gene. The other transcript is $p14^{ARF}$. The CDKN2A gene, with its two transcripts, is an important tumor suppressor gene, with a central role in the control of cell proliferation and apoptosis (Sherr, 2001). Haller at al. examined the relevance of the CDKN2A tumor suppressor pathway in GISTs and found that the low mRNA expression of the CDKN2A transcript $p16^{INK4a}$, was associated with more aggressive clinical behaviour and adverse prognosis (Haller et al., 2005).
Recently, additional insight on the biology of GISTs has recently been gained through gene microarray studies. These studies identified a number of genes whose expression is relatively increased if compared to that of other soft tissue tumors. Many genes have not been well characterized yet. Among these a GIST-specific gene, encoding for FLJ10261protein, has been named "Discovered on GIST 1" (DOG1).
DOG1 has been recently identified as a gene on human chromosome 11q13, which is amplified in esophageal cancer, bladder tumors, and breast cancer. Using immunohistochemistry and *in situ* hybridization technology with *DOG1*-specific probes, West et al., (West et al., 2004) showed DOG1 overexpression in both KIT and PDGFRα GISTs.
Because their biological function is still unknown, it is unclear why DOG1 is so widely expressed in GISTs. Two possibilities would exist. First, DOG1 might have a role in receptor kinase signal transduction pathways; second, it may be a fortuitous marker of the GIST phenotype, with no direct connection to the KIT and PDGFRα signaling pathways. The finding that mast cells are also immunoreactive for DOG1 tends to favour the former possibility (West et al., 2004). In this context, DOG1 would be considered a potential alternative therapeutic target.
p27 cell cycle inhibitor seems to be downregulated in malignant GISTs; cycle regulatory proteins (cyclins B1, D and E, cdc2, CDK2, CDK4 and CDK6), p53, pRb and cyclinA have been found to be upregulated in high-risk GISTs. The above mentioned molecules have been proposed as immunohistochemical target of high-risk gastrointestinal stromal tumors molecular (Romeo et al., 2009).

In addition to the above mentioned markers, an increasing list of prognostic factors have been reported: Ezrin, Raf kinase inhibitor protein, COX-2, bcl-2, CA II (Romeo et al. 2009). However standardized protocols for interpretation of these markers have not been establish yet.

5. GISTs epidemiology and clinical presentation

Mesenchymal tumors of GI tract are divided into two main groups: 1) tumors which are histological identical to thei soft tissue counterpart (e.g., lipomas, leiomyiomas etc.); 2) gastrointestinal stromal tumors, which represent approximatively 1% of all primitive tumors, 0.1-3% of all gastrointestinal neoplasia and are, at the same time, the most frequent mesenchimal lesions of gastrointestinal tract. GISTs have distinctive histologic and clinical features that vary according to their primary site of origin.

The exact incidence of GIST in USA and in Europe is hard to determine, since GISTs have only been recognized and diagnosed as a separate entity since the late 1990s. Recent population-based studies performed in Sweden (Nilsson et al., 2005), Holland (Goettsch et al., 2005) found incidences of approximately 14.5 and 12.7 cases/million/year, respectively. These findings would translate into an annual incidence in Europe of about 8,000-9,000 cases and in USA of about 5,000 new cases per year. They are frankly malignant in 10-30% of cases and are responsible for cancer mortality in 2% of cases. Sporadic GIST has no clear gender preference; at the time of diagnosis, the majority of patients with GISTs are between 40 and 80 years old, with a median age of 60 years.

GISTs can develop in any part of the digestive system, from the oesophagus to the rectus. They arise predominantly in the stomach (60%), jejunum and ileum (30%), duodenum (5%), and colon-rectum (<5%). Very few cases have been described in the oesophagus and appendix (<5%) (Miettinen et al., 2006). Tumor lacking any association with the bowel wall (omental, retroperitoneal and mesenteric localizations) are known as Extra Gastrointestinal Stromal Tumor (EGIST). Mesentery or omentum lack the ICCs; this fact confirms GIST's origin from these cells.

Most gastrointestinal stromal tumors occur sporadically, and present themselves as solitary lesions.

GISTs have a predominant exophytic growth, along the gastrointestinal tract and frequently protrude into the abdominal cavity. In smaller neoplasia, the mucous membrane is frequently intact, and the muscle layer of the mucosa seems to be coalescent with the muscular layer; in other cases, tumor may compresses the muscular layer, from which it is delimited by a thicker collagen band. Ulceration of mucous membrane may occur but in case of large, aggressive tumors.

Commonly, the tumors are well delimited, not encapsulated, firm in consistency, whitish. Macroscopically, GISTs present most often as a well-circumscribed and highly vascular tumors. On gross examination, these tumors appears fleshy pink or tan-white and may show hemorrhagic foci, central cystic degenerative changes, or necrosis. Invasion of the adjacent organs can occurs in one-third of cases (Figure 3).

Due to their submucosal or intramural location, small GISTs come often incidentally evident during radiological procedures, surgical intervention for other pathologies or autoptic examination. On the other hand, patients with malignant GIST often present with disseminated disease.

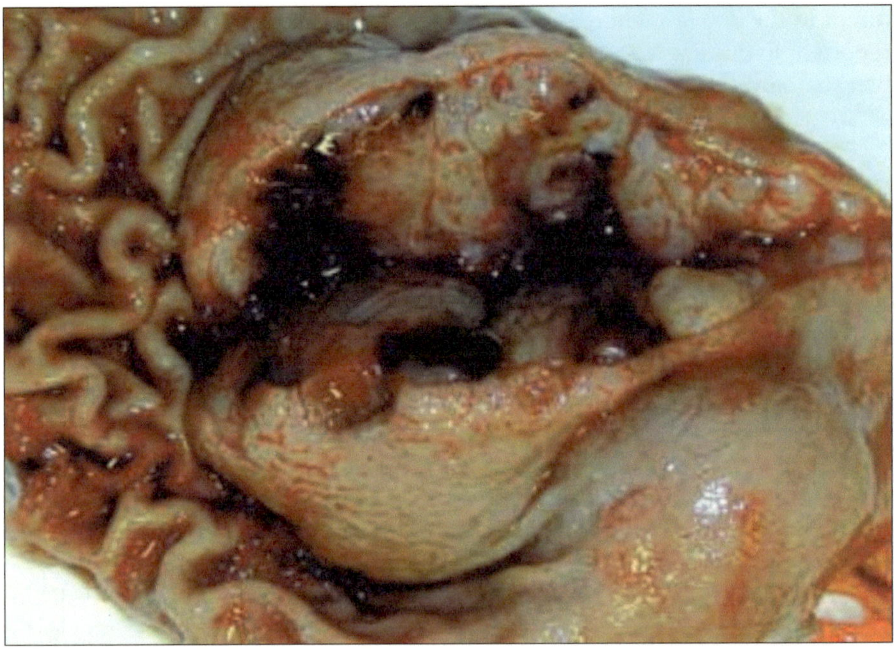

Fig. 3. Commonest macroscopic appearance of gastrointestinal stromal tumor. gelatinous cut surface with focal haemorrhagic foci, central cystic degenerative changes and/or necrosis

The presenting manifestations of gastrointestinal stromal tumors depend on the GI site of origin, the precise portion of the gut wall in which the tumor is located and the size of the neoplasia. A significant number of benign, small tumors are asymptomatic and are accidentally found. In larger tumors, clinical symptoms include abdominal pain, fatigue, dysphagia, satiety and obstruction. Patients may present with chronic acute GI bleeding (causing anemia), acute GI bleeding (caused by erosion through the gastric or the bowel mucosa), or rupture into the abdominal cavity causing intraperitoneal hemorrhage. In general, about 70% of GISTs are associated with clinical symptoms, 20% are not, and 10% are detected at autopsy (Nilsson et al., 2005). The median tumor size in each of the previous categories is 8.9, 2.7 and 3.4 cm, respectively (Nilsson et al., 2005).

In general, tumors infiltrating the mucosa are virtually always malignant. Radiologic imaging studies, including barium contrast, computer tomography and endoscopic ultrasound, are commonly used for the diagnosis and the evaluation of these neoplasms. In addition, some tumors can be diagnosed by cytology, although separation of benign and malignant GISTs is usually not always possible.

GIST metastasis have been reported in 50% of patients. They can quite often occur 10-15 years after initial surgery; therefore, long-term follow-up is required. Metastases develop primarily in the abdominal cavity and liver, exceptionally in lymph nodes or in the lung (De Matteo et al., 2000).

Most of GISTs of omentum, mesenteries, and retroperitoneum are metastatic from the GI-tract (Tsukuda et al., 2007); in these cases, peritoneal involvement with ascites may be the sole presenting features of these tumors.

Histopathologic examination of surgical resection specimens represents the most common method in GIST diagnosis.

6. Familial, paediatric and multiple GISTs

Although the majority of gastrointestinal stromal tumors present as sporadic and solitary gastrointestinal mass in adults aging 50-70 years, with no associated risk factors, a small subset of GISTs (about 5%) occur in the setting of familial or idiopathic multitumor syndrome (neurofibromatosis type 1-NF1-, Carney triad and familial GIST syndrome), in with heritable mutations in KIT or PDGFRα receptors have also been identified (Table 1).

Patients with NF1 have an up to 180-fold increased risk for GISTs, compared with the general population. The majority of NF1 GISTs arise in the small bowel, often in a multifocal appearance. In this context, distinguishing patients with NF1 and multiple GISTs from those having sporadic GISTs with multiple metastasis is often essential. Most of NF1 gastrointestinal stromal tumors are small, cytologically bland, mitotically inactive and follow and indolent course. Then the suspicious for NF1 should be high when multiple, small intestinal GISTs are encountered. Diffuse hyperplasia of ICCs is often seen in the myenteric plexus adjacent to neoplastic masses.

The pathogenesis of NF1 GISTs appears to be different from that of sporadic tumors since it has been demonstrated a very low frequency of associated KIT and PDGFRα mutations (Ponti et al., 2011).

Paediatric GISTs are considered a separate clinicopathologic entity and occur predominantly in the second decade (Juneway et al., 2007). In paediatric and adolescents, gastrointestinal stromal tumors account for 1-2% of all GISTs (Fletcher et al., 2002).

Molecular analyses detect KIT/PDGFRα mutations in a small percentage of cases of paediatric GI stromal neoplasia (10-15%) (Antonescu et al., 2006; Fletcher et al, 2002). Paediatric GISTs are more prevalent in females (female/male ratio: 9:1), occur preferentially in the stomach (88%), display epithelioid or mixed cell morphology (82%), lack of ICC hyperplasia (100%), are slow to progress but can metastasize with a worse prognosis. Unlike adult GISTs, these tumors commonly involve local lymph nodes Prakash et al., 2005). By contrast, paediatric GISTs with KIT or PDGFRα mutations have very different features: prevalence is greater in males, lesions tend to be unifocal and usually occur in extragastric locations, and spindle-cell morphology is found in all cases (Agaram et al., 2008; Janeway et al., 2007); in other words, they share many of the features of spontaneous adult tumors.

Paediatric gastric GISTs are sometimes associated with pulmonary condromas or paragangliomas, referred to as Carney triad (CT) (Carney, 1999). A number of other lesions have been described in the condition also including pheochromocytomas, oesophageal leiomyomas and adrenocortical adenomas. CT is now considered a novel form of multiple endocrine neopasia (MEN), a genetic condition with a female predilection. Stratakis et al., recently reported a deletion within the 1pcen13-q21 region, which harbours the SDHC gene. Another frequent change was the loss of 1p. although GISTs showed more frequent losses of 1p than paragangliomas, the pattern of chromosomal changes was similar in the two tumors, despite their different tissue origin and histology. These findings are consistent with a common genetic aetiology.

Another separate condition in which the dyad GISTs/paragangliomas is inherited is Carney-Stratakis syndrome (CSS); here germline mutation of SDHB, SDHC and SDHD genes (but not KIT or PDGFRα) has been found.

In very rare case, GISTs may be detected in many organs (multiple GISTs). However, this is not necessarily an indicator of greater aggressiveness. In general, multiple sporadic GISTs are associated to familial GIST syndrome, to Carney triad or Carney-Stratakis syndrome. In many cases of multiple GISTs, prognosis and treatment differ from those of conventional GISTs. In these circumstances differential diagnosis is mainly based on clinical and genetic studies, rather than on morphological, immunohistochemical or molecular analyses.

7. Pathology

Morphologic evaluation reveals three principal subtypes of GIST, depending on the cytomorphology. Most GISTs (about 70% of cases) are comprised of a fairly uniform population of spindle cells, arranged in a short fascicles or whorls; cytoplasm is sparse, fibrillary, basophilic or rarely eosinophilic, and sometimes contain PAS positive juxtanuclear vacuoles. The nuclei are monomorphous, flattened, have blunt ends and are bullet or cigar shaped; however, they can also be long and pointed. Nuclear pleomorphism is not characteristic for GISTs. The tumor may exhibit a storiform, pallisading or herringbone pattern; in this cases GISTs can simulate smooth muscle tumors or tumors of the neural sheet (Figure 4). Larger tumors may present calcification zones.

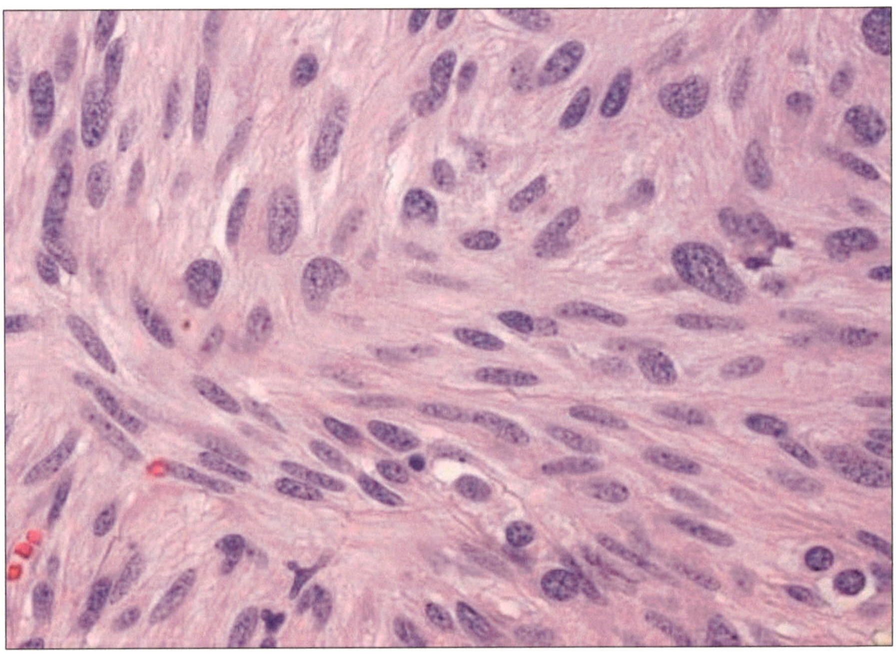

Fig. 4. Spindle cells GIST variant. Ematoxinin-Eosin staining, 20X magnification (from GIST Support International - Pathology Analyses for GIST at www.gistsupport.org).

About 20% of GISTs are dominated by epithelioid round cells, with eosinophilic to clear abundant cytoplasm, and arranged in sheets and nests (Figure 5). This microscopic form can be particularly found in gastric tumors, showing round or eccentric nuclei, with perinuclear vacuolization and small nucleoli. Scattered multinucleated giant cells or cells with bizarre nuclei can be present. Mitotic figures are rare. Collections of extracellular collagen, called skeinoid fibers, may be seen in either spindle and epithelioid variants.
In general, most epithelioid GISTs arising in the stomach are benign, in contrast with those of small intestine, where the prominent epithelioid component is often malignant (Miettinen et al., 2005).

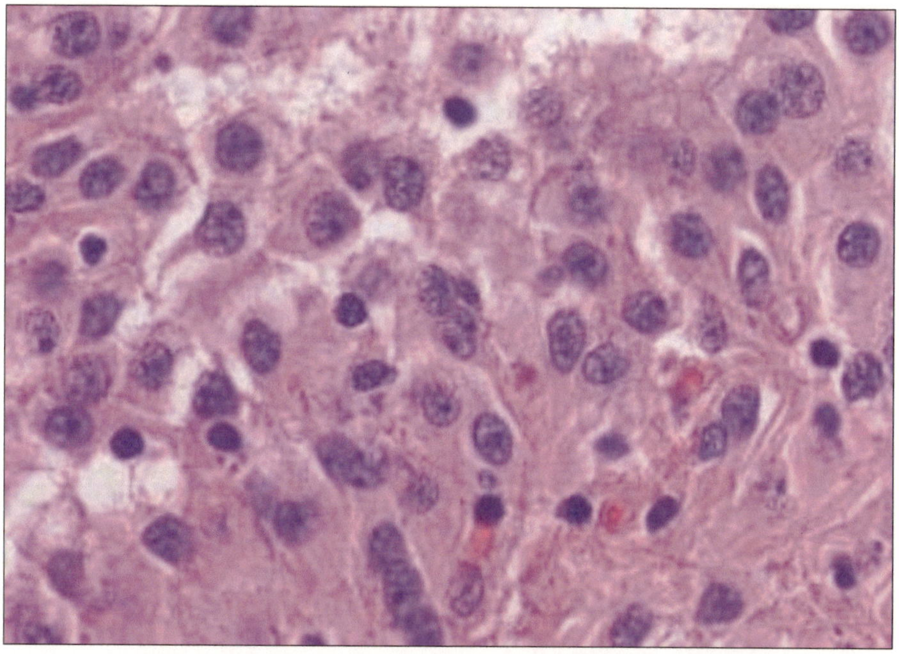

Fig. 5. Epitheliod cells GIST variant. Haematoxinin-Eosin staining, 40X magnification

Approximately 9% of gastrointestinal stromal tumors show mixed morphology, being composed of both spindle and epithelioid cells (biphasic GIST). Variable cellularity as well as sclerotic, collagenous or myxoid stromal changes can be seen. Spindle cells usually can show nuclear palisading or storiform growth pattern, resembling that of peripheral schawannomas; in these cases prominent perinuclear vacuolization is a typical feature.

Overall, GISTs are considered as uniform and monotonous tumors. Pleomorphic and dedifferentiated GISTs are occasionally seen. Mitotic activity is generally low.

Rarely, GISTs may also show signet ring cell features and oncocytic variant. The first variant frequently affect women, and present itself as a small, well circumscribed nodule, histologically characterized by a proliferation of large, round to oval cells containing abundant clear cytoplasm and with nuclear displacement toward the cellular periphery. The second histological variant is characterized by an abundance of mitochondria and by eosinophilic cytoplasm.

Gastrointestinal autonomic nerve tumor (GANT) is also considered a GIST variant. GANT main localization is the small intestine, rarely the stomach, occasionally the large intestine, the oesophagus, the retroperitoneum and the mesentery. It affects mainly the male population aged over 60 years. Tumors occurring in younger person and with gastric localization usually accompany the Carney triad. Microscopically, GANTs are similar to other stromal tumors (epithelial or spindle shape with myxoid stroma). The presence of skeinoid fibers is more frequently observed than in other stromal tumors; lymphoid aggregates can be frequently seen around the tumoral cell nests, but malignant potential is not different from that of GISTs with the same size, histological features and localization.

Although a lot of information has been reported about the histological pattern of GISTs, little is still known about the cytologic appearance of gastrointestinal stromal tumors, particularly in effusions.

In ascitic fluid, GISTs morphologically resemble adenocarcinomas (Figure 6). The most confusing findings are related to cells in a nested pattern and to the occurrence of prominent intracytoplasmic vacuoles (Figure 7). In these case, it would be essential the immunocytochemical study of the neoplasia.

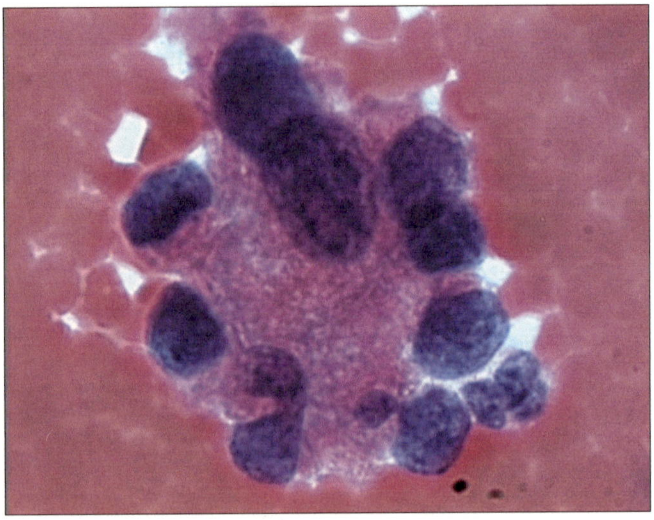

Fig. 6. Morphologic appearance of gastric GIST in ascetic fluid: 3-dimensional sheets of cells with a gland-like prevalent pattern. Papanicolaou stain, 40X magnification

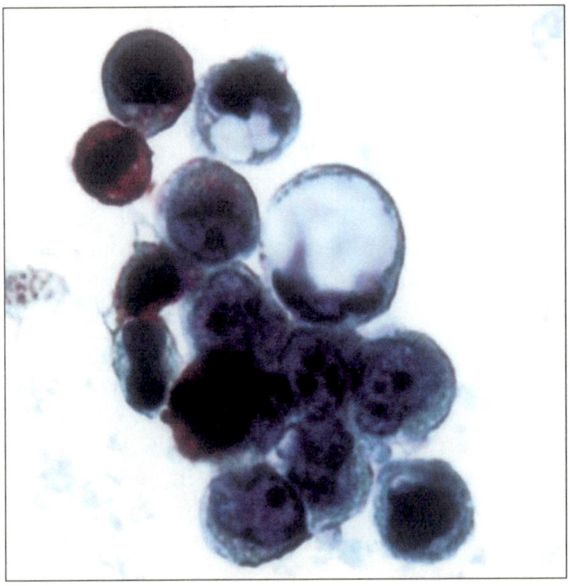

Fig. 7. Gastric GIST in ascetic fluid: tumor cells show epithelioid appearance with high nuclear/cytoplasmic ratio, prominent nucleoli and intracytoplasmic PAS-negative vacuoles, PAS stain, 63X magnification (from Zappacosta et al., (2009) Thin-Layer Cytopathology of a Gastrointestinal Stromal Tumor (GIST) in Effusion: Diagnostic Dilemmas. *Annals of Clinical & Laboratory Science*, 39; 4:367-371)

8. Morphologic risk assessment in GISTs

Although the vast majority of GISTs smaller than 2 cm are clinically benign lesions, occasionally patients will develop metastasis, sometimes 5 years or more after primary excision. Therefore, the older classification that used the terminology "benign" or "malignant" GIST have been replaced by stratification schemes which help in predicting the risk of aggressive clinical behaviour.

The first widely accepted scheme was published in 2002 by Fletcher et al., after a consensus workshop held at the National Institutes of Health (Fletcher et al., 2002). In this scheme, risk assessment is based on tumor size and mitotic activity (per 50 high power fields - HPF). The most important cut-offs as indicator of aggressive clinical behaviour is tumor size of 5 cm and 5 mitoses/50 HPF. According to this 2002 consensus guidelines, all GISTs may have malignant potential. In 2005 and 2006, Miettinen et al., from the AFIP presented two very massive studies of gastric and jejunal/ileal GISTs, providing strong evidence that tumor located in the stomach have a much lower rate of aggressive behaviour that of jejunal and ileal, having similar size and mitotic activity (Miettinen et al., 2006). Basing on these publications, anatomic location is now included as an additional parameter in risk assessment for GIST, together with nodular size and mitotic count (Table 2). To date, tumoral location outside of the stomach seems to be a prognostic factor for survival independent of the mitotic count and tumor size.

Of interest is the prognostic nomogram that could be drawn after the complete surgical resection of primary GISTs; basing on GIST size, mitotic index and site parameters, it would be useful in predicting the probability of 2- and 5-years recurrence free survival (Gold et al, 2009), and in stratifying patients for adjuvant pharmacological treatment.

Mitotic index (number of mitosis/50 HPF)	Size (cm)	Risk of progressive disease in Gastric, duodenal, small intestinal and rectal localization
≤5	≤2	None in all
≤5	>2≤5	Very low, low, low, low
≤5	>5≤10	Low, not reported, moderate, not reported
≤5	>10	Moderate, high, high, high
>5	≤2	None, nor reported, high, high
>5	>2≤5	Moderate, high, high, high
>5	>5≤10	High, nor reported, high, not reported
>5	>10	High in all

Table 2. Risk stratification of primary GIST.

8.1 Gastric GISTs

These neoplasia can be divided into four main types: benign and malignant spindle cell tumors (Figure 3) and benign and malignant epithelioid tumors (Figure 4). These tumor types can usually be distinguished by the assessment of a combination of histologic features (Tables 3 and 4)

ELEMENTS	BENIGN	MALIGNANT
Cellularity	high	high
Mitotic figures	<2/50 HPF	Usually >5/50 HPF
Perinuclear vacuoles	present	usually absent
Nuclear atypia	often absent	Present

*HPF, high power field

Table 3. Histologic characteristics of benign and malignant spindle shape gastric GIST

ELEMENTS	BENIGN	MALIGNANT
Cellularity	low	high
Mitotic figures	<2/50 HPF	Usually >5/50 HPF
Nuclear atypia	often absent	usually present
Necrosis	often absent	usually present

Table 4. Histologic characteristics of benign and malignant epithelioid gastric GIST

8.2 Small bowel GISTs

The small bowel represents the second most common site of gastrointestinal stromal tumors. Unlike GISTs of the stomach, those that occur in the small gut are usually composed of spindle cells. usually, epithelioid variants are rare. The spectrum of histologic feature is completely different from that of gastric localization (Table 5). In general, more small bowel GISTs are malignant than gastric tumors.

ELEMENTS	BENIGN	MALIGNANT
Cellularity	low	high
Mitotic figures	<5/50 HPF	>5/50 HPF
Nuclear atypia	low	high
Necrosis	absent	often present

Table 5. Histologic characteristics of small bowel stromal tumors

8.3 Colonic GISTs

The colon represents the least common site of these neoplasia. Histologically, benign stromal tumors of the colon are rare. Colonic GISTs are more heterogeneous than those of other sites and include highly cellular spindle cell tumors and highly pleomorphic sarcomas. Most patients present metastases at the time of clinical presentation and show poor survival (Miettinen at al., 2009). Tworek et al., showed that an infiltrative growth pattern in the muscolaris propria, mucosal invasion and high mitotic counts (>5/50 HPF) correlated significantly with metastasis and deaths Tworek et al., 1999). On the other hand, coagulative necrosis and dense cellularity were found to be minor criteria in the prediction of adverse outcome (Table 6)

ELEMENTS	Low-risk GISTs	High-risk GISTs
Cellularity	low	usually high
Mitotic figures	≤5/50 HPF	>5/50 HPF
necrosis	absent	usually present

Table 6. Histologic characteristics of low-risk and high-risk colonic GISTs

8.4 Anorectal GISTs

The most common mesenchymal tumor of this site is leiomyoma. This lesion is composed of differentiated benign smooth muscular cells derived from the muscolaris mucosae and is usually cured by local excision. Apart leiomyoma, most mesenchymal tumors of the anorectum are spindle cell neoplasia, having similar light microscopy, immunohistochemical and molecular genetic alterations of those of GISTs arising in other parts of GI tract. All anorectal GISTs are malignant, regardless their histologic appearance. Hovewer, several recent studies have showed the contrary. As with GISTs which develop in other sites, a wide range of features can be used to separate benign from malignant behaviour (Table 7).

ELEMENTS	Low-risk GISTs	High-risk GISTs
Tumor size	<2 cm	>5 cm
Cellularity	low	usually high
Mitotic figures	≤5/50 HPF	>5/50 HPF

Table 7. Histologic characteristics of low-risk and high-risk GISTs

The most common form of anorectal GIST develops in the muscolaris propria and is characterized by fascicles of densely cellular, spindle shaped cells with elongated and uniform nuclei, often showing prominent nuclear palisading. Unlike gastric GISTs, anorectal tumors rarely show predominant epithelioid morphology. Malignant tumors tend to be located in the muscolaris propria and show mild nuclear atypia and high mitotic counts. Tworek et al., demonstrated that tumor size larger than 5 cm and an infiltrative growth pattern within muscolaris propria, correlates with an adverse outcome (Tworek et al., 1999). On the contrary, nuclear plemorphism, necrosis, mitotic counts and intramuscular localization did not correlate with clinical behaviour. This studies also revealed a long latency period before recurrence and metastasis, thus emphasizing the need for long-term follow-up in patients with these tumors

8.5 Oesophageal GISTs

Benign leiomyiomas represents the most common type of mesenchymal tumor also in this site, while oesophageal GISTs are rare. These last usually have a male predilection, more often present with dysphagia, and typically arise in the distal oesophagus, often involving esophagogastric junction. Grossly the have a soft consistency, with a fleshy, variegated cut surface, frequently with central necrosis and cystic changes.

histologically, they are typically high cellular spindle shaped neoplasms, composed of mildly atypical nuclei and a wide range of mitotic activity. A variety of morphologic patterns may be seen, including sheets of cells, with or without nuclear palisading, myxoid change, and hyaline-like degeneration. coagulative necrosis and mucosal invasion are rare.

9. Immunohistochemistry of GISTs

9.1 c-kit and PDGFRα antibodies

The key features of GISTs is the positivity for the KIT (CD117) receptor tyrosine kinas (c-kit), observed in more than 95% of the tumors. c-kit is considered a marker with high levels of sensitivity. However, although c-kit positivity is a major defining features for GIST, it

should not be considered an absolute requirement. It is very important to point out that c-kit expression in GIST is a constitutional feature and not a consequence of mutation.
CD117 GIST positivity is often pancytoplasmic. Membrane staining is also observed in epithelioid variants (Figure 8).

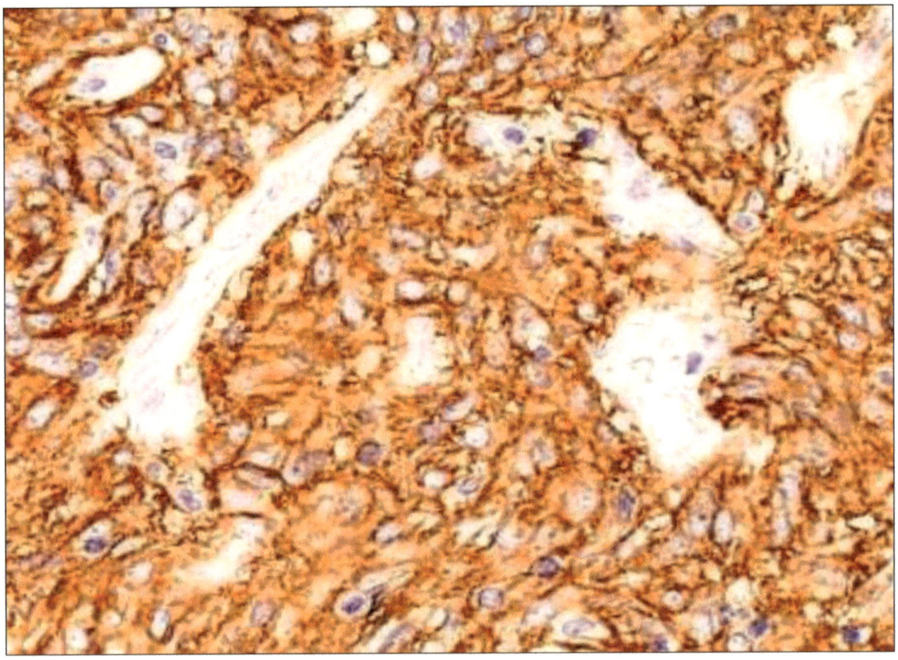

Fig. 8. CD117 GIST positivity. 20X magnification

The intensity of c-kit immunostain is variable. In most cases it is weakly and not homogeneous. In other cases, only a small percentage (10-20%) cells shows CD117 positivity. The minimum percentage of CD117-positive tumoral cells needed to establish GIST diagnosis has been not established yet but if this percentage is below 10% and positive cells are isolated or arranged in small groups it is important to differentiate them from mast cells.
There are some rare cases of negative c-kit GISTs (about 5%). In these cases, diagnosis of GIST should be cautious and should be made only after the elimination of some cases that might determined the marker negativity, such as possible technical errors. Specific kit antibodies should react with normal KIT-positive components, such as mast cells and ICC and not with normal smooth muscle cells or fibroblasts. CD117 could also tested negative in GISTs previously treated with imatinib, and in metastatic or congenital lesions. In these cases, a molecular study o KIT or PDGFRα mutations would be essential.
Basing on the above considerations, it is possible to assert that CD117 is not specific for GISTs. This marker is also expressed, in seminoma, melanoma, follicular thyroid carcinoma, small cells lung carcinoma, thymic carcinoma and thymomas, angiosarcomas, chronic myeloid leukemia, mast- cell tumors, germinal tumors etc. Fortunately, the distinction between GISTs and these other tumors can be easily made with histological observation and with the use of other more specific markers.

PDGFRα strong immunopositivity is often observed in PDGFRα mutated GISTs. However, these finding needs further evaluation.

9.2 CD34 antibody

CD34 is less sensitive than CD117 and is expressed in 60-70% of tumors localized in oesophagus, rectum, and rarely in small bowel. CD34 is a hematopoietic progenitor cell antigen also expressed in endothelial cells, subsets of fibroblasts and in tumors related to these cell types. CD34 expression does not seem to have a significant prognostic factor.

9.3 Muscle cell markers

Approximately 30% of GISTs, more often located in small intestine, are positive for smooth muscle actin (SMA), whose expression is sometimes reciprocal with that of CD34. SMA positivity may be focal or extensive.

Often, when normal smooth muscle fibers infiltrate GIST cells, the result is the presence of SMA (and Desmin) positive spindle cells within stromal stromal neoplasia; this "contamination" should not be confused with GIST SMA-positivity; in fact GIST SMA-positivity has been statistically correlated with favourable prognosis in gastric and intestinal neoplasia (Miettinen et al., 2006).

Desmin positivity is rare in GISTs of all sites, If positive to desmin, GISTs have gastric localization and are of epithelioid variant. It is important to note that imatinib treatment may induce desmin expression.

H-caldesmon it has been recently introduced among the diagnostic immunohistochemical panel for GISTs. It is a protein associated with actin, and is expressed in normal and neoplastic smooth muscle cells such as leiomyomas and leiomyosarcoma. The association of positivity for h-caldesmon, SMA and desmin would guide the diagnosis towards a smooth muscle tumor rather than towards a GIST.

9.4 Neural markers

S100 protein expression is rare in GISTs, but seems to be more common in neoplasia of small bowel than in that of stomach. In this context, S100 protein positivity seems to be an adverse prognostic factor in gastric but not in small intestinal GIST (Miettinen et al., 2006).

GISTs are also positive for nestin, a type VI intermediate filament protein that is typical of many stem cells, including those of nervous and muscular systems. Nestin is also present in GI schwannomas, this suggesting a relative low specificity for GIST diagnosis.

Gastrointestinal stromal tumors are positive for vimentin and negative for glial fibrillary acid protein (GFAP). This negativity helps to distinguish GISTs from GI schwannomas, that test GFAP positive.

Cytokeratin positivity can be also seen in GIST, especially CK18 and CK8, but not CK19 and CK20. Antibodies cocktails such as AE1/AE3 would usually give negative results.

9.5 DOG1

It has been recently realized that DOG1 is the same protein called anoctamin I or TMEM16A, known to act as calcium-activated chloride channel (Gomes-Pinilla et al., 2009).

DOG1 expression has been described in a large series of normal cell types, including ICCs, myoepithelial/basal cells in breast and prostate etc. The pattern of positivity is essentially cytoplasmic and/or membranous. DOG1 is now considered a higher sensitive marker of

GIST than CD117; about one-third of c-kit negative GISTs shows DOG1 positivity (Liegh et al., 2009) even if a small minority (at least, 1%) may be both CD117 and DOG1 negative.
It has been noted that only four GIST mimics potentially express both CD117 and DOG1: angiosarcomas, synovial sarcomas, Ewing's sarcomas and melanomas. In the above mentioned neoplasia, immunostaining for either markers is focal, whereas in GISTs is diffuse. It has been proposed that in histologically suspected GIST and in presence of diffuse c-kit and DOG1 immunopositivity, no other immunohistochemical testing would be required.
It should be take in consideration that: (i) gastrointestinal leiomyomas may shows some DOG1-positive ICCs intermingled with neoplastic smooth cells; the presence of these cells within leiomyomas raises the question if these tumors are effectively true neoplasia or, instead, nodular hyperplasia. (ii) A number of carcinomas may occasionally tested positive for DOG1; some of these neoplasia, especially adenocarcinoma, may also tested CD117-positive (West et al., 2004).

9.6 Immunocytochemical markers

As previously described, in effusions GIST cells may be acquire an epithelioid appearance characterized by nested pattern and prominent intracytoplasmic vacuoles. In order to differentiate GIST from other epithelioid and non-epitheliod neoplasms, the immunocytochemical assessment of the tumor would be imperative. Positive immunoreactivity for vimentin, but not for cytokeratins, within gland-like structures would suggest the mesenchymal nature of the tumor; PAS-negativity demonstrating the lack of mucin within cytoplasmic vacuoles can also supported the diagnosis of GIST.

10. Differential diagnosis

Obviously, differential diagnosis has been very much facilitated by immunohistochemistry, using a complete and specific panel of antibodies for mesenchymal tumors. Neoplasia with smooth muscle differentiation (leiomyiomas and leiomyosarcomas, SMA+, desmin+ but CD117- and CD34-negative) will be taken into account. Differential diagnosis also includes tumors with nervous differentiation, such as gastric schwannomas (S100+, CD117-), tumors with fibrous differentiation, such as fibromatosis (CD117-), inflammatory gastric polyps and inflammatory myofibroblastic pseudo-tumor CD117- and CD34-).
Histological pattern would exclude retroperitoneal undifferentiated liposarcomas, as well as two CD117-positive mesenchymal tumors: metastasis of malignant melanomas and angiosarcoma.
In effusion, GIST should be distinguished from mesotheliomas and amelanotic melanomas. Mesotheliomas may display PAS-negative, or rarely PAS-positive, intracytoplasmic vacuoles but, in contrast with GISTs, it shows pancytokeratin positivity. Amelanotic melanomas may show a weak CD117-positivity, as well as vimentin-positivity; however, melanomas cells usually grow as single elements and stain S100-positive, whereas GIST cells aggregate in three-dimensional clusters usually staining S100-negative.

11. GISTs surgical approach

Complete surgical resection with microscopically negative margins represents the standard of care for patients presenting primary resectable GISTs. Particularly, neo-adjuvant therapy for those with resectable disease is actually not recommended, although preoperative drug administration may be considered for patients with marginally resectable tumors and for those having potentially resectable disease but at increased risk of significant morbidity.

11.1 Lesions smaller than 2 cm

When small oesophageal, gastric or duodenal nodule less than 2 cm in size are detected, endoscopic biopsy may be difficult; in these cases, laparoscopic or laparotomic excision may be elective in order to achieve a histological diagnosis. According to the new guidelines, GISTs smaller than 2 cm must to be regarded as essentially benign. For this reason, the standard approach to these patients relies on endoscopic ultrasound assessment and then follow-up. Excision would then reserved for patients whose tumor increases in size or becomes symptomatic. For rectal tumor, the standard approach is biopsy/excision after ultrasound assessment, regardless of tumor size, because the risk of GIST at this site is high.

11.2 Lesions larger than 2 cm

In this case, the standard approach is biopsy/excision. In presence of larger mass, especially if surgery might imply multivisceral resection, multiple core needle biopsies represent the standard approach. Obviously, accurate assessment of the histotype is essential.

12. Molecular target therapy

Because constitutive activation of KIT and PDGFRα has been demonstrated in GIST development, the inhibition of these activated kinases has been verified to be effective for the treatment of this neoplasia.

Imatinib is an orally bioavailable 2-phenylaminopyrimidine derivative, developed in 1990s as a treatment for myelogenous leukemia. Imatinib shuts off oncogenic signalling from the fusion oncogene Bcr-Abl in chronic myelogenous leukemia cells by occupying the ATP-binding pocket of the Abl kinase domain. Abl shares considerable homology with the type III receptor tyrosine kinase family (Reichardt et al., 2011). In addition to the inhibitory effect of imatinib mesylate on PDGFRα and Bcr-ABL, it has been found an inhibitory effect on wild-type KIT (Reichardt et al., 2011). The fist GIST patient successfully treated with imatinib was reported in 2001 (Druker et al., 2001). Subsequently, a multicenter trial on advanced GIST was done in 2002 and significantly effect was reported (van Oosterom et al., 2002). Consequently, FDA approved imatinib mesylate as an effective therapeutic agent for patients with metastatic or un-resectable KIT-positive GIST. Obviously, an accurate pathological diagnosis of GIST condition by using immunohistochemistry for KIT is necessary.

Imatinib reliably achieves disease control in 70-85% of patients with advanced GISTs, with a median progression-free survival of 20-24 months. The estimated median overall survival time following imatinib therapy exceeds 36 months (Corless et al., 2008).

As previously described, imatinib is effective in the majority of GIST patients, but tumor regrowth by resistant clones occurs during continuous therapy (secondary resistance) (Joensuu et al., 2008). The main cause of this event seems to be a second mutation in the same genes. For these reasons, several new drugs for GIST including the imatinib-resistant are under development or clinical trials.

12.1 Therapy for localised resectable disease

Estimation of recurrence risk of GIST after resection is very important during the selection of patients for adjuvant imatinib.

Size, mitotic count and anatomic localization have been widely accepted as predictive of outcome, but tumor rupture, incomplete resection and c-kit/PDGFRα mutational status also impact on disease-free survival (Joensuu et al., 2008). Particularly, when compared with exon 11 mutants, the presence of exon 9 mutations and wild-type GIST were the strongest adverse prognostic factors for response, risk of progression and death (Dematteo et al., 2009).

Questions remain regarding post-operative or adjuvant therapy. The American College of Surgeons Oncology Group conducted a randomised, phase III trial of adjuvant imatinib after surgical resection of primary GIST. They randomly assigned 713 adults with a completely resected GIST ≥3 cm in size and immunohistochemically positive for KIT to 1 year of adjuvant imatinib or placebo. At a median follow-up of 20 months, 30 patients in the imatinib group had recurred or died, versus 70 given placebo. The 1-year recurrence free-survival was 98% versus 83%, favouring imatinib (Dematteo et al., 2009). basing of these findings, FDA approved the use of imatinib for patients having completely resected GIST ≥3 cm in size. However, the optimal duration of therapy for patients remains unclear. Actually two additional European trials have been completed: EORTC 62024 randomized trial assessing the overall survival of patients with intermediate and high-risk GIST after 2 years of imatinib or observation alone; Scandinavian Sarcoma Group trial XVIII, that evaluated recurrence-free survival of patients with high-risk disease after 1-3 years of adjuvant imatinib. Data from there trials are shortly to be published.

12.2 Therapy for un-resectable or metastatic disease

Systemic chemotherapy for advanced GIST is highly ineffective: response rate is less than 10% (Dematteo et al., 2002). Imatinib blocks KIT/PDGFRα signalling by binding to the ATP-binding pocker required for phosphorylation and activation of the receptor. In vitro data demonstrated that imatinib leads to the interruption of cell proliferation through the inhibition of downstream phosphorylation.

12.3 Management of refractory GISTs

The median time to progression on first-line imatinib is about 2-2.5 years. Dose escalation should be considered in patients who had imatinib therapy but shows clear evidence of progression. The efficacy of this approach was demonstrated in the European dose-finding study (Zalcberg et al., 2005).

Sunitinib, nilotinib and dasatinib represent the second generation of multitargeted tyrosine kinase inhibitors. The role of this new pharmacological approach to GIST was established by an international phase III trial performed on patients intolerant to or with imatinib-resistant GIST. this trial revealed highly statistically significant benefits in terms of response rate, time of progression and overall survival.

Sorafenib, is a multitargeted tyrosine kinase inhibitor with potent activity against B-RAF tyrosine kinase, VEGFR, PDGFR, KIT and FLT3. has been investigated in a phase II study involving patients with imatinib- and sunitinib-resistant GIST. This trial demonstrated an overall progression free survival of about 22 months (Wiebe et al., 2008).

Heat shock proteins (HSP) help to maintain malignant pathway buy stabilizing mutated proteins. Inhibition of HSP 90 destroys the activated KIT/ PDGFRα, potentially leading to a therapeutic effect in GIST patients. However, an international phase III trial in patients with metastatic and/or un-resectable neoplasia after failure of imatinib and sunitinib demonstrated higher mortality rate among patients in the treatment arm.

Flavopiridol is an inhibitor of cyclin-dependent kinase (CDK1 and CDK2). In preclinical studies, this molecule induced a high level of apoptosis in GIST cells, at clinical doses.

Although a wide range of studies has been done about GISTs pharmacological therapy, many questions remain controversial. For these reasons, currently sunitinib represents the only standard targeted therapy available in imatinib-refractory GISTs. For this reason, an urgent need for new drugs exist. However, due to the relatively rarity of GIST disease, it is may difficult to accumulate an adequate number of patients for clinical trials. Basing on these considerations, collaborations among medical centers worldwide would be crucial.

13. Mutational analyses to predict GISTs pharmacological response

It has been reported that also the location of KIT and PDGFRα mutations is related to pharmacological response to imatinib (Wardelmann et al., 2007). Then, assessing the presence and the type of GIST mutation can help to predict response to pharmacological therapy. Particularly, GIST with JM domain mutations of the PDGFRα appeared to respond to imatinib but GIST with TK domain mutation of the same gene, as well as GIST without any detectable c-kit or PDGFRα mutations did not. Moreover, pharmacological response to imatinib was higher for GIST with mutations with JM domain of c-kit gene than that of GIST with EC domain mutation of the same gene (Debiec-Rychter et al., 2006)..

The genotype profile associated with primary resistance to sunitinib is just the opposite of that of imatinib: KIT exon 9 mutetions and wild-type genotype predict for a better response that exon 11 mutations (Heinrich et al., 2008). Mutations predicting primary resistance to both imatinib and sunitinib, such as PDGFRα exon 18 mutation (D842V), also exist (Corless et al., 2005; Prenen et al., 2006).

In a majority of cases, secondary resistance to imatinib is due to prolonged exposure to the drug, which induces the emergence of GIST cell clones, bearing additional, resistance-mediating mutations (Liegl et al., 2008; Wardelmann et al., 2006). The vast majority of these so-called secondary mutations causing imatinib resistance have been found in KIT exons 13, 14, 17 and 18., and there are some clinical data suggesting that the exon 13 andd 14 mutations are still sensitive to sunitinib whereas mutations at exons 17 and 18 are not (Heinrich et al., 2008).

Basing on these considerations mutational analyses are considered to be a needful requirement to predict the effectiveness of pharmacological therapy on GIST patient. For these reasons, it would be of great importance the molecular classification of GISTs, which both emphasizes the molecular contest of the tumor as well as provides a quick reference for syndromes with which stromal tumors may be associated (Table 8).

GIST type	Response to pharmacological therapy
KIT mutation	
Exon 11	Excellent response to imatinib
Exon 9	Intermediate response to imatinib
Exon 13	Sensitive to imatinib in vitro
Exon 17	Sensitive to imatinib in vitro
PDGFRα mutation	
Exon 12	Sensitive to imatinib in vitro
Exon 18	D842V: poor response; other mutations are sensitive
Wild type	Poor response to imatinib

Table 8. Molecular classification of GIST (Corless CL et al., 2001, modified)

14. Methodologies to assess GISTs response to therapy

As more GISTs are being resected following down-staging with imatinib therapy, there are increasing published data regarding the pathological changes induced by such therapy, although these data are still evolving.

These changes can be divided into those representing GIST regressing with therapy and into those of GIST resistant to therapy. In the former case, the typical macroscopic appearance is a gelatinous cut surface with focal haemorrhagic and/or necrosis. Histologically, these features correspond with a hypocellular, mixoid and/or fibrotic stroma, containing scattered residual GIST cells with pyknotic nuclei and minimal cytoplasm.

When compared with its pre-treated counterpart, an imatinib regressing GIST will typically shows reduced or absent CD117 immuno-positivity, reduced CD34 positivity and a reduction of mitotic activity and Ki67 labelling index.

There is little documentation of whether GISTs demonstrating primary imatinib resistance show specific histopathological changes; by contrast, the range of pathological features associated with secondary resistance to imatinib has been more widely described.

Radiologically, secondary resistance is often characterized by re-emergence of 2-[18F]fluoro-D-glucose (FDG) uptake on positron emission tomography (PET) scan and/or peripheral thickening or nodule formation in a previously responding tumor on TC scan Mabille et al., 2009; (Mabille et al., 2009; Van den Abbeele et al., 2008). This corresponds macroscopically with one or more solid area showing the above-mentioned regressing changes within the tumor.

Some case reports described secondary resistant GISTs developing a more epithelioid appearance, with large cells containing abundant eosinophilic cytoplasm. However, there are doubts regarding the true significance of this phenomena.

Actually, overall assessment of response to therapy in patients undergoing treatment for GISTs actually relies decrease of tumor density as observed on computed tomography, since tumor progression may present as change in size or density. In this context, it has been proposed a new set of response evaluation criteria in which tumor response is defined as a 10% decreased in unidimensional tumor size or a 15% decrease in tumor density on tomography (Choi et al., 2007).

15. GISTs prognosis

Several clinical factors have been reported to define the prognosis of GISTs. Tumor tumor size, location in the fundus or gastroesophageal junction, coagulative necrosis, ulceration, mucosal invasion and mitotic count have all been identified as unfavourable factors. In addition, male sex, high age, high Ki67 (or MIB-1) grade, desmin staining and incomplete surgical resection have been also shown to be factors having a wrong impact on the overall survivals (Ozguc et al., 2005). Moreover, it seems that patients with tumor rupture have a very high risk of recurrence, since tumor rupture taking place either spontaneously or at surgery increases the risk of intra-abdominal tumoral implants. Tumor rupture seems to be independent of the size and mitotic count (Rutkowski et al., 2007; Takahashi et al., 2007).

Almost all small GISTs detected incidentally or through serial sectioning of surgical or autoptic specimens display an uniformly spindle cell morphology and are CD117+/CD34+; however, expression of CD34 is often lacking or is focal in the secondary compartment. It has been demonstrated that the secondary localization generally evolved from the corresponding lower-grade primary site through accumulation of additional chromosomal imbalances. This fact suggest that progression from low-grade to high-grade morphology, as well as eventual metastatic behaviour is driven by increasing chromosomal instability (Agaimy et al., 2009). In summary, it seems that sequential chromosomal alterations rather than KIT or PDGFRα mutations would drive the evolution to eventual GIST more aggressive behaviour (Agaimy et al., 2009). However, further studies are needed to clarify these correlations and link them to clinical outcome.

Since additional prognostic factors are continuously proposed in the medical literature, the need of accurate risk stratification becomes increasingly urgent. Accurate risk stratification is crucial for the selection of patients who are most likely to benefit from pharmacological therapy (Demetri et al., 2007).

16. Conclusions

This review provides an overview on gastrointestinal stromal tumor. Pathogenesis, morphologic evaluation, immunohistochemical markers, risk assessment, molecular analyses and therapies, represent the basic elements of the present work, as well as the disquisition regarding the pharmacological approach to this neoplasia and the mechanisms of drug resistance.

At a glance overview emerges how GISTs, from being poorly defined, treatment-resistant neoplasia become a well recognised, well understood and effectively treated neoplasia.

In this context, progresses in understanding of GIST biology laid the foundation for the fist model of target therapy. GIST model is now widely adopted in programmes focusing on a variety of other solid tumors.

17. References

Abulafia, O., Pezzullo, J.C. & Sherer, D.M. (2003). Performance of ThinPrep liquid-based cervical cytology in comparison with conventionally prepared Papanicolaou smears: a quantitative survey. *Gynecol Oncol* 90: 137-144.

Agaimy, A., Haller, F., Gunawan, B., Wünsch, P.H. & Füzesi, L. (2009). Distinct biphasic histomorphological pattern in gastrointestinal stromal tumours (GISTs) with common primary mutations but divergent molecular cytogenetic progression. *Histopathology* 54: 295-302.

Agaram, N.P., Laquaglia, M.P., Ustun, B., Guo, T., Wong, G.C. & Socci, N.D. (2008). Molecular characterization of pediatric gastrointestinal stromal tumors. *Clin Cancer Res* 14: 3204-3215.

Antonescu, C.R., Besmer, P. & Guo, T. (2005). Acquired resistance to imatinib in gastrointestinal stromal tumor occurs through secondary gene mutation. *Clin Cancer Res* 11: 4182–4190.

Antonescu, C.R. (2006). Gastrointestinal stromal tumor (GIST) pathogenesis, familial GIST, and animal models. *Semin Diagn Pathol* 23: 63–69.

Cajal, S.R. (1983). Sur les ganglions et plexus nerveux de l'intestin. *CR Soc Biol* 45: 217–23.

Carney J.A. (1999). Gastric stromal sarcoma, pulmonary chondroma, and extra-adrenal paraganglioma (Carney Triad): natural history, adrenocortical component, and possible familial occurrence. *Mayo Clin. Proc.* 74: 543–52.

Choi H., Charnsangavej C. & Faria S.C. (2007). Correlation of computed tomography and positron emission tomography in patients with metastatic gastrointestinal stromal tumor treated at a single institution with imatinib mesylate: proposal of new computed tomography response criteria. *J Clin Oncol* 25: 1753–1759.

Chompret A., Kannengiesser, C., Barrois, M., Terrier, P. & Dahan, P. (2004). PDGFRA germline mutation in a family with multiple cases of gastrointestinal stromal tumor. *Gastroenterology* 126: 318–321.

Corless, C.L., McGreevey, L., Haley, A., Town, A. & Heinrich, M.C. (2002). KIT mutations are common in incidental gastrointestinal stromal tumors one centimeter or less in size. *Am J Pathol* 160: 1567–1572.

Corless, C.L., Schroeder, A. & Griffith D. (2005). PDGFRA mutations in gastrointestinal stromal tumors: frequency, spectrum and in vitro sensitivity to imatinib. *J Clin. Oncol* 23; 5357–5364.

Corless, C.L. & Heinrich, M.C. (2008). Molecular Pathobiology of Gastrointestinal Stromal Sarcomas. *Ann Rev Pathol Mech Dis* 3: 557–586.

Debiec-Rychter, M., Cools, J. & Dumez, H. (2005). Mechanisms of resistance to imatinib mesylate in gastrointestinal stromal tumors and activity of the PKC412 inhibitor against imatinib resistant mutants. *Gastroenterology* 128: 270–279.

Debiec-Rychter, M., Sciot, R. & Le, C.A. (2006). KIT mutations and dose selection for imatinib in patients with advanced gastrointestinal stromal tumours. *Eur J Cancer* 42; 1093–1103.

DeMatteo, R.P., Lewis, J.J. & Leung, D. (2000). Two hundred gastrointestinal stromal tumors: recurrence patterns and prognostic factors for survival. *Ann Surg* 231: 51–58.

Dematteo, R.P., Heinrich, M.C. & El-Rifai, W.M. (2002). Clinical management of gastrointestinal stromal tumors: before and after STI-571. *Hum Pathol* 33: 466–477.

Dematteo, R.P., Ballman, K.V. & Antonescu, C.R. (2009). Adjuvant imatinib mesylate after resection of localised, primary gastrointestinal stromal tumour: a randomised, double-blind, placebo-controlled trial. *Lancet* 373: 1097–1104.

Demetri, G.D., Benjamin, R.S. & Blanke, C.D. (2007). NCCN Task Force report: management of patients with gastrointestinal stromal tumor (GIST)—update of the NCCN clinical practice guidelines. *J Natl Compr Canc Netw* 5(Suppl 2): S1-S29.

Druker, B.J., Talpaz, M., Resta, D.J., Peng, B., Buchdunger, E., Ford, J.M., Lydon, N.B., Kantarjian, H., Capdeville, R., Ohno-Jones, S. & Sawyers, C.L. (2001). Efficacy and safety of a specific inhibitor of the BCR-ABL tyrosine kinase in chronic myeloid leukemia. *N Engl J Med* 5; 344: 1031-1037.

Fletcher, C.D., Berman, J.J. & Corless, C. (2002). Diagnosis of gastrointestinal stromal tumors: a consensus approach. *Hum Pathol* 33: 459–465.

Haller, F., Gunawan, B. & von Heydebreck, A. (2005). Prognostic Role of E2F1 andMembers of the CDKN2A Network in Gastrointestinal Stromal Tumors. *Clin Cancer Res* 11: 6589-6597.

Furitsu, T., Tsujimura, T., Tono, T., Ikeda, H., Kitayama, H., Koshimizu, U., Sugahara, H., Butterfield, J.H., Ashman, L.K., Kanayama, Y., Matsuzawa, Y., Kitamura, Y. & Kanakura, Y. (1993). Identification of mutations in the coding sequence of the proto-oncogene c-kit in a human mast cell leukemia cell line causing ligand-independent activation of c-kit product. *J Clin Invest* 92: 1736–1744.

Goettsch, W.G., Bos, S.D. & Breekveldt-Postma, N. (2005). Incidence of gastrointestinal stromal tumours is underestimated: results of a nationwide study. *Eur J Cancer* 41: 2868–2872.

Gold, J.S., Gonen, M. & Gutierrez, A. (2009) Development and validation of a prognostic nomogram for recurrence-free survival after complete surgical resection of localised primary gastrointestinal stromal tumour: a retrospective analysis. *Lancet Oncol* 10: 1045–1052.

Gomez-Pinilla, P.J., Gibbons, S.J. & Bardsley, M.R. (2009). Ano1 is a selective marker of interstitial cells of Cajal in the human and mouse gastrointestinal tract. *Am. J Physio Gastrointest Liver Physiol* 296: 1370–1381.

Hayashi, S.I., Kunisada, M., Ogawa, M., Yamaguchi, K. & Nishikawa, S.I. (1991). Exon skipping by mutation of an authentic splice site of c-kit gene in W/W mouse. *Nucleic Acids Res* 19: 1267-1271.

Heinrich, M.C., Corless, C.L., Duensing, A., McGreevey, L., Chen, C.J., Joseph, N., Singer, S., Griffith, D.J., Haley, A., Town, A., Demetri, G.D., Fletcher, C.D. & Fletcher, J.A. (2003). PDGFRA activating mutations in gastrointestinal stromal tumors. *Science* 299: 708–710.

Heinrich, M.C., Maki, R.G. & Corless, C.L. (2008). Primary and secondary kinase genotypes correlate with the biological and clinical activity of sunitinib in imatinib-resistant gastrointestinal stromal tumor. *J Clin Oncol* 26; 5352–5359.

Hirota, S., Isozaki, K., Moriyama, Y., Hashimoto, K. & Nishida, T. (1998). Gain-of-function mutations of c-kit in human gastrointestinal stromal tumors. *Science* 279:577–80 Rubin BP, Antonescu CR, Scott-Browne JP, Comstock ML, Gu Y, et al. 2005. A knockin mouse model of gastrointestinal stromal tumor harboring kit K641E. *Cancer Res* 65: 6631–6639.

Huizinga, J.D., Thuneberg, L. & Kluppel, M. (1995). W/kit gene required for interstitial cells of Cajal and for intestinal pacemaker activity. *Nature* 373: 347–349.

Isozaki, K., Hirota, S., Nakama, A., Miyagawa, J. & Shinomura, Y. (1995). Disturbed intestinal movement, bile reflux to the stomach, and deficiency of c-kit-expressing cells in Ws/Ws mutant rats. *Gastroenterology* 109: 456–464.

Janeway, K.A., Liegl, B. & Harlow, A. (2007) Pediatric KIT wildtype and platelet-derived growth factor receptor alpha wild-type gastrointestinal stromal tumors share KIT activation but not mechanisms of genetic progression with adult gastrointestinal stromal tumors. *Cancer Res* 67: 9084–9088.

Joensuu, H. (2008). Risk stratification of patients diagnosed with gastrointestinal stromal tumor. *Hum Pathol* 39: 1411-1419.

Kang, D.Y., Park, C.K., Choi, J.S., Jin, S.Y. & Kim HJ (2007). Multiple gastrointestinal stromal tumors: clinicopathologic and genetic analysis of 12 patients. *Am J Surg Pathol* 31: 224-232.

Kindblom, L.G., Remotti, H.E., Aldenborg, F. & Meis-Kindblom, J.M. (1998). Gastrointestinal pacemaker cell tumor (GIPACT): Gastrointestinal stromal tumors show phenotypic characteristics of the interstitial cells of Cajal. *Am J Pathol* 152: 1259-1269.

Liegl, B., Kepten, I. & Le, C. (2009). Heterogeneity of kinase inhibitor resistance mechanisms in GIST. *J Pathol* 216; 64–74.

Liegl, B., Hornick, J.L., Corless, C.L. & Fletcher, C.D. Monoclonal antibody DOG1.1 shows higher sensitivity than KIT in the diagnosis of gastrointestinal stromal tumors, including unusual subtypes. *Am J Surg Pathol* 33; 437–446.

Mabille, M., Vanel, D. & Albiter, M. (2009). Follow-up of hepatic and peritoneal metastases of gastrointestinal tumors (GIST) under imatinib therapy requires different criteria of radiological evaluation (size is not everything!). *Eur J Radiol* 69; 204–208.

Maeda, H., Yamagata, A. & Nishikawa, S. (1992). Requirement of c-kit for development of intestinal pacemaker system. *Development* 116: 369–375.

Miettinen, M., El-Rifai, W., Sobin, L.H. & Lasota, J. (20029. Evaluation of malignancy and prognosis of gastrointestinal stromal tumors: a review. *Hum Pathol* 33: 478–483.

Miettinen, M., Sobin, L.H. & Lasota, J. (2005). Gastrointestinal stromal tumors of the stomach: a clinicopathologic, immunohistochemical, and molecular genetic study of 1765 cases with long-term follow-up. *Am. J Surg Pathol* 29: 52–68.

Miettinen, M., Makhlouf, H. & Sobin, L.H. (2006). Gastrointestinal stromal tumors of the jejunum and ileum: a clinicopathologic, immunohistochemical, and molecular genetic study of 906 cases before imatinib with long-term follow-up. *Am J Surg Pathol* 30: 477–489.

Miettinen, M., Sobin, L.H. & Lasota, J. (2009). True smooth muscle tumors of the small intestine: a clinicopathologic, immunhistochemical, and molecular genetic study of 25 cases. *Am J Surg Pathol* 33: 430-436.

Nilsson, B., Bumming, P. & Meis-Kindblom, J.M. (2005). Gastrointestinal stromal tumors: the incidence, prevalence,

clinical course, and prognostication in the preimatinib mesylate era-a population-based study in western Sweden. *Cancer* 103: 821–829.

O'riain, C., Corless, C.L., Heinrich, M.C., Keegan, D. & Vioreanu, M. (2005). Gastrointestinal stromal tumors: insights from a new familial GIST kindred with unusual genetic and pathologic features. *Am. J Surg Pathol* 29: 1680–1683.

Ozguc, H., Yilmazlar, T., Yerci, O., Soylu, R., Tumay, V & Filiz, G. (2005). Analysis of prognostic and immunohistochemical factors in gastrointestinal stromal tumors with malignant potential. *J Gastrointest Surg* 9: 418–429

Ponti, G., Losi, L., Martorana, D., Priola, M., Boni, E., Pollio, A., Neri, T.M. & Seidenari, S. (2011). Clinico-pathological and biomolecular findings in Italian patients with multiple cutaneous neurofibromas. *Hered Cancer Clin Pract* 12; 6-9.

Prakash, S., Sarran, L., Socci, N., DeMatteo, R.P. & Eisenstat, J. (2005). Gastrointestinal stromal tumors in children and young adults: a clinicopathologic, molecular, and genomic study of 15 cases and review of the literature. *J Pediatr Hematol Oncol* 27: 179–187.

Prenen, H., Cools, J. & Mentens, N. (2006). Efficacy of the kinase inhibitor SU11248 against gastrointestinal stromal tumor mutants refractory to imatinib mesylate. *Clin Cancer Res* 12; 2622–2627.

Reichardt, P., Reichardt, A. & Pink, D. (2011). Molecular targeted therapy of gastrointestinal stromal tumors. *Curr Cancer Drug Targets* 11: 688-697.

Ricci, R., Arena, V. & Castri, F. (2004). Role of p16/INK4a in gastrointestinal stromal tumor progression. *Am J Clin Pathol* 122: 35-43.

Romeo, S., Debiec-Rychter, M. & Van Glabbeke, M. (2009). Cell cycle/apoptosis molecule expression correlates with imatinib response in patients with advanced gastrointestinal stromal tumors. *Clin Cancer Res* 15: 4191–4198.

Ronnstrand L. (2004). Signal transduction via the stem cell factor receptor/c-Kit. *Cell Mol Life Sci* 61: 2535–2548.

Rutkowski, P., Nowecki, Z.I. & Michej, W. (2007). Risk criteria and prognostic factors for predicting recurrences after resection of primary gastrointestinal stromal tumor. *Ann Surg Oncol* 14: 2018-2027.

Sabah, M., Cummins, R., Leader, M. & Kay, E. 82004). Loss of heterozygosity of chromosome 9p and loss of p16INK4A expression are associated with malignant gastrointestinal stromal tumors. *Mod Pathol* 17: 1364 -1371.

Schneider-Stock, R., Boltze, C. & Lasota, J. (20039. High prognostic value of p16INK4 alterations in gastrointestinal stromal tumors. *J Clin Oncol* 21: 1688-1697.

Schneider-Stock, R., Boltze, C. & Lasota, J. (2005). Loss of p16 protein defines high-risk patients with gastrointestinal stromal tumors: a tissue microarray study. *Clin Cancer Res* 11: 638-645.

Sherr, C.J. (2001). The INK4a/ARF network in tumour suppression. *Nat RevMol Cell Biol* 2: 731-737.

Takahashi, T., Nakajima, K. & Nishitani, A. 82007). An enhanced risk-group stratification system for more practical prognostication of clinically malignant gastrointestinal stromal tumors. *Int J Clin Oncol* 12: 369-374.

Taniguchi, M., Nishida, T., Hirota, S., Isozaki, K., Ito, T., Nomura, T., Matsuda, H. & Kitmura, Y. (1999). Effect of c-*kit* mutation on prognosis of gastrointestinal stromal tumors. *Cancer Res* 59: 4297–4300.

Torihashi, S., Ward, S.M. & Sanders, K.M. (1997). Development of c-kitpositive cells and the onset of electrical rhythmicity in murine small intestine. *Gastroenterology* 12: 144–155.

Tsukuda, K., Hirai, R., Miyake, T., Takagi, S., Ikeda, E., Kunitomo, T. & Tsuji, H. (2007) The outcome of gastrointestinal stromal tumors (GISTs) after a surgical resection in our institute. *Surg Today* 37: 953-957.

Tworek, J.A., Goldblum, J.R., Weiss, S.W., Greenson, J.K. & Appelman, H.D. (1999). Stromal tumors of the abdominal colon: a clinicopathologic study of 20 cases. *Am J Surg Pathol* 23: 937-945.

Ullrich, A. & Schlessinger, J. (1990). Signal transduction by receptors with tyrosine kinase activity. *Cell* 61: 203–212.

Van den Abbeele, A.D. (2008). The lessons of GIST-PET and PET / CT: a new paradigm for imaging. *Oncologist* 13: 8–13.

van Oosterom, A.T., Judson, I.R., Verweij, J., Stroobants, S., Dumez, H., Donato di Paola, E., Sciot, R., Van Glabbeke, M., Dimitrijevic, S. & Nielsen, O.S. (2002). European Organisation for Research and Treatment of Cancer Soft Tissue and Bone Sarcoma Group. Update of phase I study of imatinib (STI571) in advanced soft tissue sarcomas and gastrointestinal stromal tumors: a report of the EORTC Soft Tissue and Bone Sarcoma Group. *Eur J Cancer* 38 Suppl 5: S83-587.

Wakai, T., Kanda, T., Hirota, S., Ohashi, A., Shirai, Y. & Hatakeyama, K. (2004). Late resistance to imatinib therapy associated with a second KIT mutation in metastatic gastrointestinal stromal tumour. *Br J Cancer* 90: 2059–2061.

Wardelmann, E., Merkelbach-Bruse, S. & Pauls, K. (2006). Polyclonal evolution of multiple secondary KIT mutations in gastrointestinal stromal tumors under treatment with imatinib mesylate. *Clin Cancer Res* 12: 1743–1749.

Wardelmann, E., Merkelbach-Bruse, S., Büttner, R. & Schildhaus, H.U. (2007). Activating mutations in receptor tyrosine kinases with relevance for treatment of gastrointestinal stromal tumors. *Verh Dtsch Ges Pathol* 91: 165-168.

West, R.B., Corless, C.L., Chen, X., Rubin, B.P., Subramanian, S., Montgomery, K., Zhu, S., Ball, C.A., Nielsen, T.O., Patel , R., Goldblum, J.R., Brown, P.O., Heinrich, M.C. & van de Rijn, M. (2004). The novel marker, DOG1, is expressed ubiquitously in gastrointestinal stromal tumors irrespective of KIT or PDGFRA mutation status. *Am J Pathol* 165: 107-113.

Wiebe, L., Kasza, K.E. & Maki, R.G. (2008). Activity of sorafenib (SOR) in patients (pts) with imatinib (IM) and sunitinib (SU)-resistant (RES) gastrointestinal stromal tumors (GIST): a phase II trial of the University of Chicago Phase II consortium. *J Clin Oncol* 26:553-557.

Zalcberg, J.R., Verweij, J. & Casali, P.G. (2005). Outcome of patients with advanced gastro-intestinal stromal tumours crossing over to a daily imatinib dose of 800 mg after progression on 400 mg. *Eur J Cancer* 41: 1751–1757.

Zhang, Z., Zhang, R., Joachimiak, A., Schlessinger, J. & Kong, X..P. (2000). Crystal structure of human stem cell factor: implication for stem cell factor receptor dimerization and activation. *Proc Natl Acad Sci USA* 97: 7732–7737.

2

Treatment Options for Gastrointestinal Stromal Tumors

Kai-Hsi Hsu
Institute of Clinical Medicine, College of Medicine, National Cheng Kung University
Department of Surgery, Tainan Hospital, Department of Health, Executive Yuan, Tainan
Taiwan, Republic of China

1. Introduction

The term gastrointestinal stromal tumor (GIST) in the description of a specific group of gastrointestinal nonepithelial tumors lacking the microscopic evidence of smooth muscle or characteristics of neural immunoreactivity was first introduced by Mazur and Clark (Mazur & Clark, 1983). The common origin of GIST and interstitial cell of Cajal (ICC), the pacemaker cells in the digestive tract, was proposed due to their immunohistochemical and ultrastructural similarities. The definition of GISTs as tumors originating from ICC was further confirmed according to the findings that both GIST and ICC express KIT and that most GISTs have gain-of-function mutations of *KIT*, the proto-oncogene that encodes a 145 kDa transmembrane tyrosine kinase KIT receptor. Mutation of different exons of the *KIT* oncogene results in activation of the tyrosine kinase activity of KIT, leading to ligand-independent kinase activity and uncontrolled cell proliferation as well as resistance to apoptosis (Demetri et al., 2002; Hirota et al., 1998; Kindblom et al., 1998; Savage & Antman, 2002). More than 90% of GIST have constitutive activation of the KIT protein as a result of *KIT* mutation and in GIST without KIT mutations, gain-of-function of platelet derived growth factor receptor α (PDGFRA) are present in about one-third of cases. It was recently proposed that ETV1, one of the ETS family transcription factor, can be a lineage survival factor that cooperates with KIT in gastrointestinal stromal tumours. GIST arises from ICCs with high levels of endogenous ETV1 expression that, when coupled with an activating KIT mutation, drives an oncogenic ETS transcriptional program (Chi et al., 2010; Roberts & Eisenberg, 2002; Rubin et al., 2001).

GIST was estimated to occur in about 14.5 cases per million and was the most common mesenchymal tumor of the gastrointestinal tract. The most common locations of GIST are the stomach (50-60%), small intestine (20-30%), colon and rectum (10%), and esophagus (5%). Patients mostly present with nonspecific symptoms and signs (69%) and initial metastasis was noted in about 15-50% of GISTs (DeMatteo et al., 2000; Fletcher et al., 2002; Nilsson et al., 2005; Roberts & Eisenberg, 2002; Shinomura et al., 2005).

The accurate diagnosis of GIST should be based on tumor morphology and immunohistochemistry. GIST tumors grossly appear as well-defined submucosal lesion with prominent vasculature and occasional hemorrhage or ulceration (Fig. 1A and 1B.). Under morphologic examination in the immunohistochemical analysis, GIST tumor cells are generally classified as three morphologic subtypes, including spindle cell type in the majority, epithelioid cell type and mixed type composed of both spindle and epithelioid cells (Fig. 1C). Similarly, tumor cells in GIST cell lines *in vivo* presents as spindle cell morphology in the majority, regardless of the types of the GIST cell line (Fig. 1D).

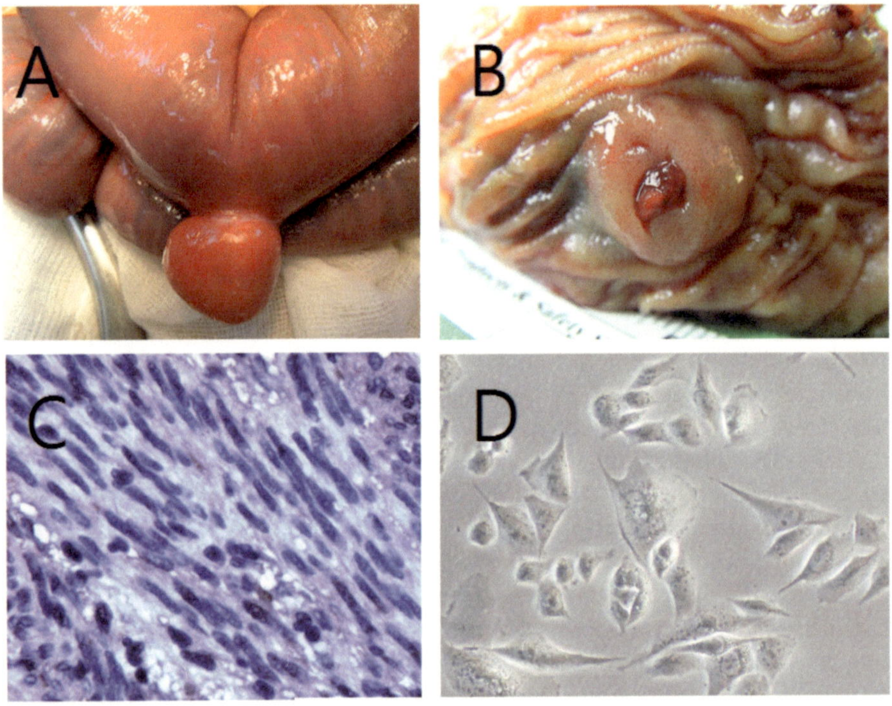

Fig. 1. Macroscopic and microscopic inspection of GIST tumor.
A. Small intestinal GIST. B. GIST tumor with central ulceration. C. GIST tumor cell by immunohistochemical staining demonstrating both types of spindle and epithelioid tumor cells. D. GIST tumor cell line.

In the diagnosis of GIST, KIT has been shown to be a specific and sensitive marker in the differential diagnosis of gastrointestinal mesenchymal tumors. The majority of GISTs express KIT, and approximately only 4-5% of GISTs are KIT negative. There may be different KIT-staining patterns KIT-negative GISTs preferentially occur in the stomach and usually show pure epithelioid or mixed cytomorphology (Debiec-Rychter M ei al., 2004; Hirota et al., 1998; Kindblom et al., 1998; Medeiros et al., 2004).

In recent years, numerous antibodies for the diagnosis of GIST have been identified. These immunohistochemical markers were mainly noted and verified in molecular studies and may be of value in the diagnosis in KIT-negative GISTs. Discovered on GIST (DOG1), an up-regulated transmembrane protein found in GISTs, is one of the markers of significance. Recent studies have demonstrated that antibodies against DOG1 have greater sensitivity and specificity than KIT (CD117) and CD34, serving as specific immunohistochemical markers for GIST regardless of the KIT/PDGFRA mutation or KIT immunohistochemical expression. Carbonic anhydrase II (CA II) and protein kinase C (PKC)-theta, a member of the protein kinase C family, in addition to being biomarkers frequently expressed in the majority of GISTs with high specificity, are also of diagnostic as well as prognostic values (Blay et al., 2004; Duensing et al., 2004; Espinosa et al., 2008; Lee et al., 2008; Liegl et al., 2009; Miettinen et al., 2009; Parkkila et al., 2010; West, RB et al., 2004).

The role of biopsy in the diagnosis of GIST is unclear. In tumors with fragile consistency and hypervascularity, biopsy is not suggested due to risk of bleeding, capsular perforation with rupture and tumor seeding. Although tissue biopsy can be conducted safely and accurately by endoscopy or other image-guided methods, the submucosal location of the tumors often make accurate sampling difficult. Necrosis, ulceration and hemorrhage are common in GIST tumor tissues and may limit and preclude the feasibility and plausibility of fine needle aspirates or core biopsies. In certain situations, biopsies may be of value in differential diagnosis when other disease entities are suspected or when diagnosis is necessary for subsequent planning of treatment (Garcia dePolavieja et al., 2010)

Imaging studies play a diagnostic role for evaluation of suspected GIST patients for characterization of the tumor. Contrast-enhanced computerized tomography (CT) scanning and occasionally magnetic resonance imaging (MRI) are the imaging modality of choice for initial evaluation and [^{18}F]2-fluoro-2-deoxy-D-glucose-positron emission tomography (FDG-PET)/CT has recently become important in both diagnosis and assessment of tumor response to targeted therapy in the adjuvant as well as neoadjuvant therapy in GIST.

For small tumors found incidentally, CT scanning or endoscopic ultrasound is recommended (Blackstein et al., 2006; Van den Abbeele et al., 2008).

While the treatment of GISTs with radiotherapy or systemic chemotherapy was unsuccessful in the majority, complete surgical resection remains the gold standard in the management of primary GIST. The recurrence rate of GIST, even in patients with resectable GIST, ranges from 17 to 24% in some series but chas also been reported to be as high as 80%. The median survival for patients with recurrence is about 9-12 months (Demetri et al., 2002; Iesalnieks et al., 2005; Nilsson et al., 2005 ; Shinomura et al., 2005; Zhu et al., 2010).

Imatinib mesylate, an tyrosine kinase inhibitor (TKI) for both normal and mutated KIT found in most GISTs, was the first effective drug in the treatment of metastatic GIST and was approved by the Food and Drug Administration (FDA) for the treatment of unresectable and metastatic GIST in 2002 (Kwon et al., 2001; DeMatteo et al., 2002; Demetri et al., 2002; Savage & Antman, 2002). Adjuvant therapy with imatinib theoretically might improve the curative rate after complete resection of primary GIST by eradicating residual microscopic disease. Trials on adjuvant imatinib after complete resection of primary GIST have been evaluated in patients with a substantial risk of relapse. Recent studies confirmed that adjuvant target therapy with imatinib was effective in improving disease-free survival in GIST after surgery in high-risk patients , potentiating upcoming wide clinical application of adjuvant imatinib treatment in GIST. Since the introduction of imatinib as the target therapy for treatment of advanced GIST, acquired or secondary resistance to imatinib was found to develop in some GIST patients (Corless et al., 2004; Dematteo et al., 2009; Demetri et al., 2002; Heinrich & Corless, 2005; Verweij et al., 2004). Another tyrosine kinase inhibitor, sunitinib malate has recently been approved as a second-line treatment for GIST patients who develop resistance to or cannot tolerate imatinib. Sunitinib has also been approved by the US FDA as second-line therapy for patients with advanced GIST. Newer agents are currently being evaluated in clinical trials. Identifying factors or biomarkers predicting high risk of disease progression in GIST patients thus becomes increasingly important and has been reported in numerous studies (Blanke et al., 2009; Corless et al., 2004; Keun et al., 2008). Numerous studies have been devoted to the identification of specific clinical and pathological markers of prognostic significance (Hsu et al., 2007a, 2007b, 2010a, 2010b; Kwon et al., 2001; Miettinen et al., 2002; Rudolph et al., 1998 ; Yan et al., 2003). Among miscellaneous prognostic parameters, tumor size and mitotic figure have been considered most useful and reliable predictive variables for prognosis with good reproducibility and statistical consistency. A Consensus guidelines and classification system for GIST risk stratification, referred to as the National Institutes of Health (NIH) Consensus Criteria for GIST risk stratification, that categorizes GIST patients with GIST into low, intermediate, and high-risk groups according to these two parameters has been proposed and was widely applied in the clinical setting for risk analysis for patients with GIST (Hsu et al., 2007a, 2007b; Fletcher et al., Shinomura et al., 2005).

Recently, the integration of tumor locationas the third parameter in NIH Consensus Criteria for GIST risk stratification, with intestinal localization of the tumor being a poor prognostic factor, was proposed to help more accurately predicting risk of recurrence and poor prognosis after surgery in patients with GIST, so that potential candidates for adjuvant imatinib therapy can be identified (Gold et al., 2009; Joensuu, 2008; Patel, 2011).

With the advent and rapid progress in the development as well as application of TKI in GIST, the treatment of GIST evolves significantly in recent years. Adjuvant, neoadjuvant therapy and new TKI agents are among the most focused issues of intensive investigations in the management of GIST in the post-TKI era. Revolutionary innovations in surgical techniques such as newly developed laparoscopic modalities have also contributed to the armamentarium of GIST management. Treatment options for GIST with respect to disease stages and different intervention strategies will be presented in this chapter.

2. Primary resectable GIST

2.1 General principles of surgery

Surgical resection has been the standard treatment for patients with localized, resectable GISTs. Specific surgical strategies are required according to the organ involved, tumor location, and tumor size. The goal of resection is to achieve complete (R0) excision of the tumor with negative margins, in the absence of residual disease grossly and microscopically. In general, primary GIST tumors tend not to invade surrounding organs or tissues. Wedge or segmental resection of the involved organs or tissues bearing the tumor is adequate. Lymph node metastasis is uncommon and lymphadenectomy has been considered unnecessary in GIST. In rare occasions when enlarged nodes are found at the time of operation, these should be removed with the primary GIST tumor. It is generally acceptable that a margin of 2 cm be adequate. However, there are no prospectively collected data available with regard to the adequate margin and to whether the extent of resection margins correlate with the risk of tumor recurrence or metastasis.

During operation, care should be taken to thoroughly evaluate the peritoneal cavity, especially the liver and peritoneum, the most common sites of disease spread for metastasis. Suspicious peritoneal lesions should be resected. Extreme care should also be taken during manipulation of the tumor to prevent excessive bleeding and peritoneal dissemination of tumor cells so that tumor rupture, one of the contributing factors associated with recurrence, does not happen.

Before the TKI era, surgery was the only curative and effective treatment for GISTs. Recemt studies have proved that adjuvant imatinib can delay recurrence and improve survival in selected patients with high-risk GIST. In patients with advanced or metastatic GIST, imatinib is the standard treatment, wiht surgery of residual masses being an option. Preoperative imatinib is an emerging and promising treatment of choice for patients with initially unresectable GIST. Such neoadjuvant therapy offers the chance of converting or reduction of the unresectable GIST into resectable diseases.

2.2 Surgery in relation to tumor location

2.2.1 Gastric GIST

The stomach is the most common tumor location for GISTs. Patients often present with GI bleeding or obstruction. Their diagnosis and are usually made by endoscopy and endoscopic ultrasound that identifies the intramural origin of the tumor. Biopsy occasionally may of help in the diagnosis of GIST. Small tumors are occasionally found during endoscopy for other indications and endoscopic resection when feasible may be indicated. Surgical intervention is necessary for gastric GIST not amenable to endoscopic resection and depends primarily on the location and size of the tumor within the stomach. As with all GISTs, the principle operative treatment is complete resection with negative margins. Special care should be taken to prevent potential tumor rupture by meticulously manipulating the tumor during the operation. The location of GIST in the lower third of the stomach may be a favorable factor, however, the exact significance of different tumor sites for prognosis of gastric GISTs needs to be further clarified. Most would advocate a distal gastrectomy with Billroth I or II reconstruction in tumor of considerable sizes. Proximal lesions on the lesser curve orlocalization close to the gastroesophageal junction may be difficult to surgical resection, especially in tumors with large-sized or wide base. In tumors that become adherent to adjacent structures, en bloc excision with omentectomy, splenectomy, or distal pancreatectomy may be indicated to ensure capsule integrity as well as R0 resection. Unlike gastric cancer, omentectomy or lymphadenectomy is not necessary unless the presence of involvement by intraoperative evaluation (Gervaz et al., 2009; Huang et al., 2010; Miettinen et al., 2005; Privette et al., 2008; Silberhumer et al., 2009).

2.2.2 Small intestinal GIST

The incidence of GIST originating from the small intestine is secondary to that of gastric GIST. Small intestinal GIST of duodenal origin is rare with the incidence of less than 5%. While a majority of patients present with bleeding, large tumors can lead to GI obstruction. The best modality for diagnosis of duodenal GIST is endoscopy. Similar to gastric GIST, the operation depends on the size and location of the primary tumor as well as distance from the ampulla. One recent study showed that type of operation was not correlated to operative risk and disease recurrence, limited operation rather than more radical pancreaticoduodenectomy should be attempted whenever possible for duodenal GIST without involvement of papilla of Vater to preserve more pancreas parenchyma, duodenum, and common bile duct (Chung et al., 2010; Miettinen et al., 2003; Yang et al., 2009).

Intestinal GIST other than duodenal origin can be difficult to diagnose. CT or capsule endoscopy are optional tools in diagnosis. In this disease entity, there is a higher proportion of lesions found in the jejunum than the ileum. The same surgical principles of negative margins and prevention of tumor rupture apply equally to intestinal GISTs, regardless of the tumor location. This is best accomplished by segmental small bowel resection with primary anastomosis. As mentioned earlier, intestinal location was an independent predictor of recurrence and poor prognosis (Dematteo et al., 2008; Miettinen et al., 2005, 2006).

2.2.3 Colorectal GIST

Reports regarding GIST of colon and rectal origin have been limited in number due to its rarity. Surgical consideration of these colorectal GISTs is the same as that mention in GIST of other locations and may include local exicision or radical resection. However, for rectal GISTs, its rarity makes it difficult to assess the role of the extension of the surgical resection of the tumor. Colonic GISTs are typically treated with segmental resection and primary anastomosis. Unlike colon cancer, formal lymphadenectomy is not necessary unless obvious nodal involvement is present. Resection of rectal GISTs is more difficult and is often associated with increased rate of complication. A formal mesorectal excision is unnecessary and often leads to increased morbidity. One study retrospectively analyzed clinical characteristics of surgically treated gastrointestinal stromal tumors of the colon and rectum and demonstrates that the majority of colorectal GISTs are high-risk. Patients with high-risk colorectal GISTs have a significant likelihood of developing metastases that is associated with poor prognosis. These patients need to be closely followed for an extended period and should be considered for adjuvant therapy with tyrosine kinase inhibitors. Since rectal GISTs are often advanced, the role of neoadjuvant Imatinib in rectal GIST has also been evaluated. It has been proposed that preoperative Imatinib therapy can contribute to reduction of the size in large rectal GISTs, improving the chances of successful radical surgery and therefore decreasing the risk of morbidity and mortality (Hassan et al., 2006; Hou et al., 2009; Machlenkin et al., 2010; Mandalà et al., 2007).

2.3 Endoscopic resection

Small GIST lesions are often found incidentally during endoscopy or laparotomy for specific indications. The diagnosis of GIST is often made after endoscopic ultrasound (EUS) referral for the evaluation of submucosal lesions. Its diagnostic yield can vary. It can be as low as 68.7% without tissue acquisition and as high as 84% with tissue acquisition (Scarpa et al., 2008). When GISTs are accidentally found during routine endoscopy, decision-making may be difficult because of the lack of data regarding biology behavior, invasiveness and metastatic potential of these tumors. Endoscopic features are unable to predict tumor behavior reliably. Once a diagnosis of GIST is confirmed and metastatic disease excluded, subsequent surgical intervention should take into consideration the size and location of the tumor. Treatment of small lesions incidentally found during endoscopy, imaging studies, or surgical exploration for other indications remains controversial. It is agreed that small tumors identified at the time of laparotomy or laparoscopy be removed whenever possible without increasing the risk of tumor rupture or risk of complication such as perforation or hemorrhage. A reasonable strategy can include close follow-up and surveillance in 6–12 months. For lesions more than 2 cm in size, surgical resection is the principle treatment and is the only curative treatment of choice. Endoscopic ligation and resection shows promise as a safe and feasible technique to treat small EUS-suspected gastric GISTs (Casali et al., 2010).

2.4 Minimally invasive surgery

The role of laparoscopic approaches in the surgical management of GIST has gained increasing popularity due to the technical advantage of complete resections in a minimally invasive manner. With appropriate handling of the tumor, laparoscopic surgery has been proved safe and effective in selected patients. Laparoscopy is particularly being used with increasing frequency for GIST originating from the stomach. Laparoscopic resection of gastric GISTs appears technically feasible and is associated with favorable outcomes. It is generally agreed that tumors up to 5 cm can be safely approached laparoscopically. It is also important to follow the same surgical principles of laparotomy when performing laparoscopic GIST resections, including complete R0 resection with free margins, avoidance of accidental tumor rupture intraoperatively, and use of a retrieval bag to prevent spillage and seeding of tumor cells into the peritoneum. While there has been no prospective randomized trial directly comparing laparoscopic and open approaches for gastric GIST, several retrospective series have demonstrated that the laparoscopic approach is associated with low morbidity, mortality, and satisfactory oncologic results. Laparoscopic surgery can be conducted in combination with intra-operative endoscopic assistances according to tumor size and location. Innovative techniques in laparoscopic surgery, including single-port laparoscopic surgery or incisionless surgical approach such as natural orifice transluminal endoscopic surgery (NOTES), have been applied in clinical practice in recent years. These surgical approaches have been reported to be associated with significantly fewer complications, reduced pain, faster recovery, and improved cosmesis compared with traditional open or laparoscopic approaches. It is likely that these newly developed minimally invasive surgery will be applied to miscellaneous surgical diseases, including GIST, in the near future (Catena et al., 2008; Choi et al., 2007; Horgan et al., 2011; Karakousis et al., 2011; Kingham & DeMatteo, 2009; Novitsky et al., 2006; Otani et al., 2006; Privette et al., 2008; Sasaki et al., 2010; Sexton et al., 2008Woodall et al., 2009).

2.5 Adjuvant therapy

The success of IM in the treatment of metastatic GIST and the significant risk of recurrence of GIST in the pre-TKI era with surgery alone stimulated investigation of complete surgical resection in combination with TKI treatment as adjuvant intent. The efficacy of standard dose adjuvant imatinib mesylate (400 mg/day) has been evaluated in clinical trials. The American College of Surgeons Oncology Group (ACOSOG) sponsored two randomized, double-blind, placebo-controlled studies evaluating adjuvant imatinib in completely resected, localized primary GIST. Based on the positive results from these clinical trials, the US FDA approved 400 mg/day imatinib mesylate tablets for oral use for the adjuvant treatment of adult patients following complete gross resection of gastrointestinal stromal tumor (GIST) with tumors larger than 3 cm on December 19, 2008 (DeMatteo et al., 2009). Several studies reported similar outcomes demonstrating that imatinib used in the adjuvant therapy improved recurrence-free survival significantly (Essat & Cooper, 2011). The duration of adjuvant therapy remains controversial and was not specified in the Food and Drug Administration approval since the rate of recurrences in the imatinib mesylate treated group seemed to increase at 18 months from surgery which corresponded to 6 months after discontinuing the study drug. Similar times to progression were also noted after treatment interruptions in patients with metastatic disease.New trials for evaluation of optimal duration for adjuvant therapy are currently undergoing that includes two large European trials aimed to clarify and evaluate the adjuvant duration: the Scandinavian Sarcoma Group (SSG) and the German Arbeitgemeinschaft Internistische Onkologie (AIO) are jointly conducting a randomized, phase III trial (SSGXVIII/AIO) to evaluate 1 year versus 3 years of adjuvant imatinib mesylate, inhigh-risk GIST patients. The European Organization for Research and Treatment of Cancer (EORTC) 62024 study compares adjuvant therapy for 2 years with observation (Blay et al., 2007).

3. Recurrent GIST

Surgery is the mainstay of treatment for primary resectable GISTs when there is no evidence of metastases or advanced diseases. Although surgery is the only known potentially curative treatment for primary resectable or marginally resectable GISTs, 40–90% of surgically treated patients experience disease recurrence despite complete surgical resection according to the literature. Five-year recurrence-free and disease-free survival rates of 49% and 65%, respectively, have been reported for patients undergoing complete resection. Prevention or identification of risk factors associated with increased rate of recurrence thus become one important issue in the surgical treatment of GIST (Hassan et al., 2008; Rossi et al., 2003; Singer et al., 2002).

Although it is clear that rupture of GIST tumor at operation carries a high risk of tumor recurrence, appropriate surgical management options and the associated outcomes in patients with a ruptured GIST is not clarified. One recent report showed that the risk of recurrence approaches nearly 100% in patients with GIST that ruptured into the abdominal cavity before or during operation and the associated recurrence-free survival was less than 1 year, emphasizing the necessity of adjuvant therapy in these group of high-risk patient. Another study investigates long-term follow-up of the imatinib mesylate treatment in patients with GIST would experience tumor recurrence or metastasis after radical resection and found that the imatinib mesylate treatment could prolong the survival of the patients who have recurrent GIST after the radical surgery (Zhu et al., 2010).

4. Advanced/metastatic GIST and targeted therapy

Initial metastasis can be present in about 15-50% of GIST patients (DeMatteo et al., 2000; Roberts & Eisenberg., 2002; Shinomura et al., 2005). Treatment guidelines for GIST all recognize imatinib as the standard of care for patients with advanced, unresectable, and metastatic GISTs. Imatinib mesylate has been proven to play a significant role in the treatment of advanced/metastatic GIST and has been considered the standard first line therapy in this patient group. Prognosis of patients with advanced disease improved significantly following the approval of imatinib mesylate in 2001 by FDA for this indication. The overall survival can be improved significantly in patients with advanced GIST. Patients who develop resistance to or are intolerant of first-line imatinib mesylate are commonly treated with sunitinib malate, a multi-targeted tyrosine kinase inhibitor approved by the FDA in January 2006 as second-line therapy in this disease (Blanke et al., 2008; Casali et al., 2009; Demetri et al., 2000, 2002, 2006; Nishida et al., 2008).

In the majority of patients with advanced, unresectable or metastatic GIST receiving imatinib treatment shows variable response. Response to treatment can be evaluated on CT scan as reduction of the tumor size or as decreased FDG uptake on a PET/CT scan. In the minority of cases, tumor progression develops within the first 6 months in spite of treatment, refered to as primary resistance, and in a subset of patients, the tumor may remain unchanged despite treatment. Secondary resistance is defined as situations when patients with initially good response or stable disease develop tumor progression after 12-36 months of treatment. Molecular mechanisms responsible for primary resistance differ from those of secondary resistance. *KIT* exon 9 and *PDGFRA* mutations more commonly are associated with primary imatinib resistance when compared to *KIT* exon 11 mutations. Secondary resistance is most commonly related to secondary mutations in the KIT kinase domain (Gajiwala et al., 2009; Heinrich et al., 2006, 2008; Liegl et al., 2008).

The success and significant effects of imatinib mesylate and sunitinib malate in their clinical application have led to miscellaneous investigations on a wide variety of new TKI for their potential roles in the treatment of GIST, including Nilotinib, Sorafenib, Masitinib (AB1010), Vatalanib (PTK787/ZK 222584). The majority of these multi-targeted tyrosine kinase inhibitors are designed as novel or third-line agents for treatment in imatinib-resistant GIST or imatinib and sunitinib-resistant GIST. If proved of their efficacy against GIST in currently clinical trials, these novel TKI agents will bring about a new TKI era and will definitely hold promise for future targeted therapy in GISTs (Guo et al., 2007; Joensuu et al., 2011; Le Cesne et al., 2010; Prenen et al., 2006; Sawaki et al., 2011).

5. Neoadjuvant therapy

Neoadjuvant, or downsizing treatment, defined as surgical resection for patients with previously unresectable GISTs after treatment with imatinib or other TKI, is indicated for reduction of tumor volume and for eradicating potential microscopically metastatic tumor cells prior to surgery. The rationale for neoadjuvant imatinib is based on the elimination of microscopic and metastatic disease, with additional benefits of preoperative cytoreduction of tumors, facilitating complete resection and function-sparing surgical procedures, offering selected patients with initially unresectable diseases chances of resectability and operability. In addition, if a significant response of tumor to such neoadjuvant therapy can be achieved, the risk of tumor rupture during surgical manipulation, and thus the potential of post-operative recurrence, can also be reduced theoretically.

Neoadjuvant therapy should be individualized and is indicated for patients with large tumors where resection would cause undo morbidity or functional deficit, and small tumors in difficult to treat areas such as the gastroesophageal junction or low rectum. Retrospective reports and prospective investigations evaluating the efficacy of imatinib in the neoadjuvant therapy for GIST have demonstrated promising results in terms of cytoreduction and facilitating conservative, organ-preserving surgery, as well as survival and prognostic benefits (Abhyankar & Nair, 2008; Andtbacka et al.,2007; Blesius et al., 2011; DeMatteo et al., 2007; Eisenberg et al., 2009; Fiore et al., 2009; Sjölund et al., 2010).

As a general, neoadjuvant imatinib should be considered if surgery could result in significant morbidity or loss of organ function, and subsequent surgery may be considered 4 to 12 months later after maximal tumor size reduction. Similar to adjuvant therapy, it remains relatively controversial as to the optimal duration of neoadjuvant therapy as well as the optimal timing of surgical intervention in this particular group of GIST patients. It is proposed that he timing of the surgical procedure can be critical in that resection should be conducted upon maximal response of the tumor to neoadjuvant imatinib before the development of tumor progression. The majority of patients with advanced GIST reach a response within 6 months of neoadjuvant therapy, with a median time to response of 3 months. In patients with GIST responding to neoadjuvant therapy, the time interval before potential resection should not be less than 3 months. Patients can be followed closely with serial CT scans to assess and document progressive reduction of the tumor size (Gold & DeMatteo, 2006, 2007).

PET scan is of importance in the neoadjuvant therapy for GIST in its role as an early and sensitive imaging tool for evaluation of the response of GIST to neoadjuvant treatment in the clinically setting. PET scans can help document tumor activity if the biologic effect of imitinab is unclear clinically. Response of the tumor can be detected and determined by PET after a week or less of neoadjuvant treatment and precedes CT response by several weeks. This could be of great value in patients with unresectable and advanced GIST, for which timely and accurate assessment of tumor response to adjuvant treatment is imperative to subsequent surgical strategies (Bumming et al.,2003; Dimitrakopoulou-Strauss et al., 2007; Katz et al., 2004; Lo et al., 2005; Loughrey et al., 2005; Raut & DeMatteo, 2008; Rutkowski et al., 2006; Shah et al., 2005; Stroobants et al., 2003; Yoon & Tanabe, 2007).

It may be a matter of time when neoadjuvant therapy, like adjuvant therapy, becomes standard treatment of choice in selected GIST patients with advanced or initially unresectable diseases if the optimal duration of treatment in both adjuvant and neoadjuvant therapy can be documented and substantiated.

6. Conclusion

The management of human malignancies, including GIST, requires a multidisciplinary team approach. In primary resectable GIST, the standard treatment remains surgery, which takes into consideration tumor location and tumor size in preoperative assessment. Innovation and evolvement in surgical techniques in the treatment of GIST should always accompany the general surgical principle of complete resection with negative margin and meticulous manipulation of tumor without rupture. The success of targeted therapy with imatinib mesylate in the treatment of advanced/metastatic GIST has revolutionized the management of GIST: in addition to emerging clinical investigations evaluating the effects of novel tyrosine kinase inhibitors in GIST, the significant role of imatinib mesylate and other tyrosine kinase inhibitors in the adjuvant and neoadjuvant therapy in different GIST patient groups has been proved and substantiated. The importance of adjuvant as well as neoadjuvant therapy in the management of GIST will continue to be emphasized and verified. It is likely that future treatment in GIST will move toward individualized targeted therapy in combination with surgery in order to optimize clinical outcomes including improved survival, reduced risk of recurrence and better quality of life.

7. References

Siegwart, R. (2001). Indirect Manipulation of a Sphere on a Flat Disk Using Force Information. *International Journal of Advanced Robotic Systems,* Vol.6, No.4, (December 2009), pp. 12-16, ISSN 1729-8806

Abhyankar, SA. (2008). Highlighting the role of FDG PET scan in early response assessment of gastrointestinal stromal tumor treated with imatinib mesylate. *Clinical Nuclear Medicine,* Vol.33, No.3, (March 2008), pp. 213-214, ISSN 0363-9762

Andtbacka, RH. (2007). Surgical resection of gastrointestinal stromal tumors after treatment with imatinib. *Annals of Surgery Oncology*, Vol.14, No.1, (January 2007), pp. 14–24, ISSN 1068-9265

Blackstein, ME. (2006). Gastrointestinal stromal tumours: consensus statement on diagnosis and treatment. *Canadian Journal of Gastroenterology*, Vol20, No.3, (March 2006), pp.157-163, ISSN 0835-7900

Blanke, CD (2009). Biomarkers in GIST: partly ready for prime-time use. *Clinical Cancer Research*, Vol.15, No.18, (September 2009), pp. 5603-5605, ISSN 1078-0432

Blanke, CD. (2008). Phase III randomized, intergroup trial assessing imatinib mesylate at two dose levels in patients with unresectable or metastatic gastrointestinal stromal tumors expressing the kit receptor tyrosine kinase: S0033. *Journal of Clinical Oncology*, Vol.16, No.4, (February 2008), pp. 626-632, ISSN 0732-183X

Blay, JY. (2007). Prospective multicentric randomized phase III study of imatinib in patients with advanced gastrointestinal stromal tumors comparing interruption versus continuation of treatment beyond 1 year: the French Sarcoma Group. *Journal of Clinical Oncology*, Vol.25, No.9, (March 2007), pp. 1107-1113, ISSN 0732-183X

Blay, P. (2004). Protein kinase C theta is highly expressed in gastrointestinal stromal tumors but not in other mesenchymal neoplasias. *Clinical Cancer Research*, Vol.10, No12, (June 2004), pp. 4089–4095, ISSN 1078-0432

Blesius, A. (2011). Neoadjuvant imatinib in patients with locally advanced non metastatic GIST in the prospective BFR14 trial. *BMC cancer*, Vol.15, No.11, (February 2011), pp. 72, ISSN 1471-2407

Bumming, P. (2003). Neoadjuvant, adjuvant and palliative treatment of gastrointestinal stromal tumours (GIST) with imatinib: a centre-based study of 17 patients. *British Journal of Cancer*, Vol.89, No.3, (August 2003), pp. 460–464, ISSN 0007-0920

Casali, PG. (2010). Gastrointestinal stromal tumours: ESMO clinical recommendations for diagnosis, treatment and follow-up. *Annals of Oncology*, Vol.21, Suppl.5, (May 2010), pp. 64–67, ISSN 0923-7534

Catena, F. (2008). Laparoscopic treatment of gastric GIST: report of 21 cases and literature's review. *Journal of Gastrointestinal Surgery*, Vol.12, No.3, (March 2008), pp. 561–568, ISSN 1091-255X

Chi, P. (2010). ETV1 is a lineage survival factor that cooperates with KIT in gastrointestinal

Choi, SM. (2007). Laparoscopic wedge resection for gastric GIST: long-term follow- up results. *European Journal of Surgical Oncology*, Vol.33, No.4, (May 2007), pp. 444–447, ISSN 0748-7983

Chung, JC. (2010). Surgery for gastrointestinal stromal tumors of the duodenum. *Annals of Surgical Oncology*, Vol.14, No.5, (May 2010), pp. 880-883, ISSN 1091-255X

Corless, CL. (2004). Biology of gastrointestinal stromal tumors. *Journal of Clinical Oncology*, Vol.22, No.18, (September 2004) , pp. 3813-3825, ISSN 0732-183X

Debiec-Rychter, M. (2004). Gastrointestinalstromal tumours (GISTs) negative for KIT (CD117 antigen) immunoreactivity. *Journal of Pathology*, Vol.202, No.4, (April 2004), pp. 430–438, ISSN 0022-3417

DeMatteo, RP. (2000). Two hundred gastrointestinal stromal tumors: recurrence patterns and prognostic factors for survival. *Annals of Surgery*, Vol.231, No.1, (January 2000), pp. 51-58, ISSN 0003-4932

DeMatteo, RP. (2007). Results of tyrosine kinase inhibitor therapy followed by surgical resection for metastatic gastrointestinal stromal tumor. *Annals of Surgery*, Vol.245, No.3, (March 2007), pp. 347–352, ISSN 0003-4932

Dematteo, RP. (2008). Tumor mitotic rate, size, and location independently predict recurrence after resection of primary gastrointestinal stromal tumor (GIST). *Cancer*, Vol.112, No.3, (February 2008), pp. 608–615, ISSN 0008-543X

Dematteo, RP. (2009). Adjuvant imatinib mesylate after resection of localised, primary gastrointestinal stromal tumour: a randomised, double-blind, placebo-controlled trial. *Lancet*, Vol.373, No.9669, (March 2009), pp. 1097-104, ISSN 0140-6736

Demetri, GD. (2002). Efficacy and safety of imatinib mesylate in advanced gastrointestinal stromal tumors. *New England Journal of Medicien*, Vol347, No.7, (August 2002), pp. 472-480, ISSN 0028-4793

Demetri, GD. (2006). Efficacy and safety of sunitinib in patients with advanced gastrointestinal stromal tumour after failure of imatinib: a randomised controlled trial. *Lancet*, Vol.368, No.9544, (October 2006), pp. 1329-1338, ISSN 0140-6736

Dimitrakopoulou-Strauss, A. (2007). 68 Ga-labeled bombesin studies in patients with gastrointestinal stromal tumors: comparison with 18F-FDG. *Journal of Nuclear Medicine*, Vol.48, No.8, (August 2007), pp. 1245-1250, ISSN 0161-5505

Duensing, A. (2004). Protein kinase C theta (PKCtheta) expression and constitutive activation in gastrointestinal stromal tumors (GISTs). *Cancer Research*, Vol.64, No.15, (August 2004), pp. 5127–5131, ISSN 0008-5472

Eisenberg, BL. (2009). Phase II trial of neoadjuvant/adjuvant imatinib mesylate (IM) for advanced primary and metastatic/recurrent operable gastrointestinal stromal tumor (GIST): Early results of RTOG 0132/ACRIN 6665. *Journal of Surgical Oncology*, Vol.99, No.1, (January 2009), pp. 42-47, ISSN 0022-4790

Espinosa, I. (2008). A novel monoclonal antibody against DOG1 is a sensitive and specific marker for gastrointestinal stromal tumors. *American Journal of Surgical Pathology*, Vol.32, No.2, (February 2008), pp. 210–218, ISSN 0147-5185

Essat, M. (2011). Imatinib as adjuvant therapy for gastrointestinal stromal tumors- a systematic review. *International Journal of Cancer*, Vol.128, No.9, (May 2011), pp. 2202-2214, ISSN 0020-7136

Fiore, M. (2009). Preoperative imatinib mesylate for unresectable or locally advanced primary gastrointestinal stromal tumors (GIST). *European Journal of Surgical Oncology*, Vol.35, No.7, (Ju;y 2009), pp. 739–745, ISSN 0748-7983

Fletcher, CD. (2002). Diagnosis of gastrointestinal stromal tumors: A consensus approach. *Human Pathology*, Vol.33, No.5, (May 2002), pp. 459-465, ISSN 0046-8177

Gajiwala, KS. (2009). KIT kinase mutants show unique mechanisms of drug resistance to imatinib and sunitinib in gastrointestinal stromal tumor patients. *Proceedings of the National Academy of Sciences of the United States of America*, Vol.106, No.5, (February 2009), pp. 1542–1547, ISSN 0027-8424

Garcia dePolavieja, (2010). Gastrointestinal stromal tumours at present: An approach to burning questions. *Clinical Translational Oncology*, Vol.12, No.2, (February 2010), pp. 100–112, ISSN 1699-048X

Gervaz, P. (2009). Surgical management of gastrointestinal stromal tumours. *British Journal of Surgery*, Vol.96, No.6, (February 2009), pp. 567–578, ISSN 0007-1323

Gold, JS. (2006). Combined surgical and molecular therapy: the gastrointestinal stromal tumor model. *Annals of Surgery,* Vol.244, No.2, (August 2006), pp. 176–184, ISSN 0003-4932

Gold, JS. (2007). Neoadjuvant therapy for gastrointestinal stromal tumor (GIST): racing against resistance. *Annals of Surgery Oncology,* Vol.14, No.4, (April 2007), pp. 1247–1248, ISSN 1068-9265

Gold, JS. (2009). Development and validation of a prognostic nomogram for recurrence-free survival after complete surgical resection of localized primary gastrointestinal stromal tumour: a retrospective analysis. *Lancet Oncology,* Vol.10, No.11, (November 2009), pp.1045-1052, ISSN 1470-2045

Guo, T. (2007). Sorafenib inhibits the imatinib-resistant KITT670I gatekeeper mutation in gastrointestinal stromal tumor. *Clinical Cancer Research,* Vol.13, No.16, (Auguet 2007), pp. 4874-4881, ISSN 1078-0432

Hassan, I. (2006).Clinical, pathologic, and immunohistochemical characteristics of gastrointestinal stromal tumors of the colon and rectum: implications for surgical management and adjuvant therapies. *Disease of Colon and Rectum,* Vol.49, No.5, (May 2006), pp. 609-615 ISSN 0012-3706

Hassan, I. (2008). Surgically managed gastrointestinal stromal tumors: a comparative and prognostic analysis. *Annals of Surgery Oncology*, Vol. 15, No.1, (January 2008), pp. 52-59, ISSN 1068-9265

Heinrich, MC. (2005). Gastric GI stromal tumors (GISTs): the role of surgery in the era of targeted therapy. *Journal of Surgical Oncology*, Vol.90, No.3, (June 2005), pp. 195-207, ISSN 0022-4790

Heinrich, MC. (2006). Molecular correlates of imatinib resistance in gastrointestinal stromal tumors. *Journal of Clinical Oncology*, Vol.24, No.29, (October 2006), pp. 4764–4774, ISSN 0732-183X

Heinrich, MC. (2008). Primary and secondary kinase genotypes correlate with the biological and clinical activity of sunitinib in imatinib-resistant gastrointestinal stromal tumor. *Journal of Clinical Oncology*, Vol.26, No.33, (November 2008), pp. 5352-5359, ISSN 0732-183X

Hirota, S. (1998). Gain-of-function mutations of c-KIT in human gastrointestinal stromal tumors. *Science*, Vol.279, No.5350, (January 1998), pp. 577-580, ISSN 0036-8075

Horgan, S. (2011). Clinical experience with a multifunctional, flexible surgery system for endolumenal, single-port, and NOTES procedures. *Surgical Endoscopy*, Vol 25, No.2, (February 2011), pp. 586-592, 0930-2794

Hou, YY. (2009). Imatinib mesylate neoadjuvant treatment for rectal malignant gastrointestinal stromal tumor. *World Journal of Gastroenterol*ogy, Vol.15, No.15, (April 2009), pp. 1910-1913, ISSN 1007-9327

Hsu, KH. (2007a). Significance of CD44 expression in gastrointestinal stromal tumors in relation to disease progression and survival. *World Journal of Surgery*, Vol.31, No.7, (July 2007),pp. 1438-1444, ISSN 0364-2313

Hsu, KH. (2007b). Tumor size is a major determinant of recurrence in patients with resectable gastrointestinal stromal tumor. *American Journal of Surgery*, Vol.194, No.2, (August 2007), pp. 148-152, ISSN 0002-9610

Hsu, KH. (2010a). Clinical implication and mitotic effect of CD44 cleavage in relation to osteopontin/CD44 interaction and dysregulated cell cycle protein in gastrointestinal stromal tumor. *Annals of Surgery Oncology*, Vol.17, No.8, (August 2010), pp. 2199-2212, ISSN 1068-9265

Hsu, KH. (2010b). Osteopontin expression is an independent adverse prognostic factor in resectable gastrointestinal stromal tumor and its interaction with CD44 promotes tumor proliferation. *Annals of Surgery Oncology*, Vol.17, No.11, (November 2010), pp, 3043-3052, ISSN 1068-9265

Huang, H. (2010). Different sites and prognoses of gastrointestinal stromal tumors of the stomach- report of 187 cases. *World Journal of Surgery*, Vol.34, No.7, (July 2010), pp. 1523-1533, , ISSN 0364-2313

Iesalnieks, I. (2005). Factors associated with disease progression in patients with gastrointestinal stromal tumors in the pre-imatinib era. *American Journal of Clinical Pathology*, Vol124, No.5, (November 2005), pp. 740-748, ISSN 0002-9173

Joensuu, H. (2008). Risk stratification of patients diagnosed with gastrointestinal stromal tumor. *Human Pathology*, Vol.39, No.10, (October 2008), pp. 1411-1419, ISSN 0046-8177

Joensuu, H. (2011). Vatalanib for metastatic GIST resistant to imatinib-final results of a phase II study. *British Jornal of Cancer*, Vol.104, No.11, (May 2011), pp. 1686-1690, ISSN 0007-0920

Karakousis, GC. (2011). Laparoscopic Versus Open Gastric Resections for Primary Gastrointestinal Stromal Tumors (GISTs): A Size-Matched Comparison. Annals of Surgical Oncology, Vol.18, No.6, (June 2011), pp. 1599-1605, ISSN 1068-9265

Katz, D. (2004). Neoadjuvant imatinib for unresectable gastrointestinal stromal tumor. *Anticancer Drugs*, Vol.15, No.6, (July 2004), pp. 599-602, ISSN 0959-4973

Keun, PC. (2008). Prognostic stratification of high-risk gastrointestinal stromal tumors in the era of targeted therapy. *Annals of Surgery*, Vol.247, No.6, (June 2008), pp. 1011-1018, ISSN 0003-4932

Kindblom, LG. (1998). Gastrointestinal pacemaker cell tumor (GIPACT). Gastrointestinal stromal tumors show phenotypic characteristics of the interstitial cells of Cajal. *American Journal of Pathology*, Vol.152, No.5, (May 1998), pp. 1259-1269, ISSN 0002-9440

Kingham, TP. (2009). Multidisciplinary treatment of gastrointestinal stromal tumors. *Surgical Clinics of North America*, Vol.243, No.6, (February 2009), pp. 217–233, ISSN 0039-6109

Kwon, SJ. (2001). Surgery and prognostic factors for gastric stromal tumor. *World Journal of Surgery*, Vol.25, No.3, (March 2001), pp. 290-295, ISSN 0364-2313

Le Cesne, A. (2010). Phase II study of oral masitinib mesilate in imatinib-naïve patients with locally advanced or metastatic gastro-intestinal stromal tumour (GIST). *European Journal of Cancer*, Vol.46, No.8, (May 2010), pp. 1344-1351, ISSN 0959-8049

Lee, HE. (2008). Characteristics of KIT negative gastrointestinal stromal tumours and diagnostic utility of protein kinase C theta immunostaining. *Journal of Clinical Pathology*, Vol.61, No.6, (June 2008), pp. 722–729, ISSN 0021-9746

Liegl, B. (2008). Heterogeneity of kinase inhibitor resistance mechanisms in GIST. *Journal of Pathology*, Vol.216, No.1, (September 2008), pp. 64–74, ISSN 0022-3417

Liegl, Bl. (2009). Monoclonal antibody DOG 1.1 shows higher sensitivity than KIT in the diagnosis of Gastrointestinal stromal tumors, including unusual subtypes. *American*

Journal of Surgical Pathology, Vol. 33, No.3, (March 2009), pp. 437–446, ISSN 0147-5185

Lo, SS. (2005). Neoadjuvant imatinib in gastrointestinal stromal tumor of the rectum: report of a case. *Disease of Colon and Rectum*, Vol.48, No.6, (June 2005), pp. 1316-1319, ISSN 0012-3706

Loughrey, MB. (2005). Gastrointestinal stromal tumour treated with neoadjuvant imatinib. *Journal of Clinical Pathology*, Vol.58, No.7, (July 2005), pp. 779–781, ISSN 0021-9746

Machlenkin, S. (2010). The effect of neoadjuvant Imatinib therapy on rectal gastrointestinal stromal tumours outcome and survival. *Colorectal Disease*, (October 2010), doi: 10.1111/j.1463-1318.2010.02442.x. [Epub ahead of print]

Mandalà, M. (2007). Neoadjuvant Imatinib in a locally advanced gastrointestinal stromal tumour (GIST) of the rectum: a rare case of two GISTs within a family without a familial GIST syndrome. *European Journal of Gastroenterology and Hepatology*, Vol .19, No.8, (August 2007), pp. 711-713, ISSN 0954-691X

Mazur, MT. (1983). Gastric stromal tumors. Reappraisal of histogenesis. *American Journal of Surgical Pathology*, Vol.7, No.4, (September 1983), pp. 507-519. ISSN 0147-5185

Medeiros, F. (2004). KIT-negative gastrointestinal stromal tumors: proof of concept and therapeutic implications. *American Journal of Surgical Pathology*, Vol.28, No.7, (July 2004), pp. 889–894, ISSN 0147-5185

Miettinen, M. (2002). Pathology and diagnostic criteria of gastrointestinal stromal tumors (GISTs): A review. *European Journal of Cancer*, Vol.38, Suppl.5, (September 2002), pp.39-51, ISSN 0959-8049

Miettinen, M. (2003). Gastrointestinal stromal tumors, intramural leiomyomas, and leiomyosarcomas in the duodenum: A clinicopathologic, immunohistochemical, and molecular genetic study of 167 cases. *American Journal of Surgical Pathology*, Vol.27, No.5, (May 2003), pp. 625–641, ISSN 0147-5185

Miettinen, M. (2005). Gastrointestinal stromal tumors of the stomach: A clinicopathologic, immunohistochemical, and molecular genetic study of 1765 cases with long-term follow-up. *American Journal of Surgical Pathology*, Vol.29, No.1, (January 2005), pp. 52–68, ISSN 0147-5185

Miettinen, M. (2006). Gastrointestinal stromal tumors of the jejunum and ileum: A clinicopathologic, immunohistochemical, and molecular genetic study of 906 cases before imatinib with long-term follow-up. *American Journal of Surgical Pathology*, Vol.30, No.4, (April 2006), pp. 477–489, ISSN 0147-5185

Miettinen, M. (2009). DOG1 antibody in the differential diagnosis of gastrointestinal stromal tumors: a study of 1,840 cases. *American Journal of Surgical Pathology*, Vol.33, No.9, (September 2009), pp. 1401–1408, ISSN 0147-5185

Nilsson, B. (2005). Gastrointestinal stromal tumors: the incidence, prevalence, clinical course, and prognostication in the preimatinib mesylate era–a population-based study in western Sweden. *Cancer*, Vol.103, No.4, (February 2005), pp. 821-829, ISSN 0008-543X

Nishida, T. (2008). Clinical practice guidelines for gastrointestinal stromal tumor (GIST) in Japan: English version. *International Journal of Clinical Oncology*, Vol.26, No.4, (February 2008), pp. 416–430, ISSN 0732-183X

Novitsky, YW. (2006). Long-term outcomes of laparoscopic resection of gastric gastrointestinal stromal tumors. *Annals of Surgery,* Vol.243, No.6, (June 2006), pp.:738–745, ISSN 0003-4932

Otani, Y. (2006). Operative indications for relatively small (2–5 cm) gastrointestinal stromal tumor of the stomach based on analysis of 60 operated cases. *Surgery,* Vol.139, No.4, (April 2006), pp. 484–492, ISSN 0039-6060

Parkkila, S. (2010). Carbonic anhydrase II. A novel biomarker for gastrointestinal stromal tumors. *Modern Pathology,* Vol.23, No.5, (May 2010), pp 743-750, ISSN 0893-3952

Patel, S. (2011). Navigating Risk Stratification Systems for the Management of Patients With GIST. *Annals of Surgical Oncology,* Vol.18, No.6, (June 2011), pp. 1698-704, ISSN 1068-9265

Prenen, H. (2006). Cellular uptake of the tyrosine kinase inhibitors imatinib and AMN107 in gastrointestinal stromal tumor cell lines. *Pharmacology,* Vol.77, No.1, (2006), pp. 11-16, ISSN 0031-7012

Privette, A. (2008). Laparoscopic approaches to resection of suspected gastric gastrointestinal stromal tumors based on tumor location. *Surgical Endoscopy,* Vol.22, No.2, (February 2008), pp. 487–494, ISSN 0930-2794

Raut, CP. (2008). Prognostic factors for primary GIST: Prime time for personalized therapy? *Annals of Surgery Oncology,* Vol.15, No.1, (January 2008), pp. 4-6, ISSN 1068-9265

Roberts, PJ. (2002). Clinical presentation of gastrointestinal stromal tumors and treatment of operable disease. *European Journal of Cancer,* Vol.38, Suppl.5, (September 2002), pp. 37-38, ISSN 0959-8049

Rossi, CR. (2003). Gastrointestinal stromal tumors: From a surgical to a molecular approach. *International Journal of Cancer,* Vol.107, No.2, (November 2003), pp. 171-176, ISSN 0020-7136

Rubin, BP. (2001). KIT activation is a ubiquitous feature of gastrointestinal stromal tumors. *Cancer Research,* Vol.61, No.22, (November 2001), pp. 8118-8121, ISSN 0008-5472

Rudolph, P. (1998). Immunophenotype, proliferation, DNA-ploidy, and biological behavior of gastrointestinal stromal tumors: a multivariate clinicopathological study. *Human Pathology,* Vol. 29, No.8, (August 1998), pp.791-800, ISSN 0046-8177

Rutkowski, P. (2006). Surgical treatment of patients with initially inoperable and/or metastatic gastrointestinal stromal tumors (GIST) during therapy with imatinib mesylate. *Journal of Surgical Oncology,* Vol.93, No.4, (March 2006), pp. 304-311, ISSN. 0022-4790

Sasaki, A. (2010). Tailored laparoscopic resection for suspected gastric gastrointestinal stromal tumors. *Surgery,* Vol.147, No.4, (April 2010), pp. 516-520, ISSN 0039-6060

Sawaki, A. (2011). Phase 2 study of nilotinib as third-line therapy for patients with gastrointestinal stromal tumor. *Cancer,* (March 2011), doi: 10.1002/cncr.26120. [Epub ahead of print], ISSN 0008-543X

Scarpa, M. (2008). A systematic review on the clinical diagnosis of gastrointestinal stromal tumors. *Journal of Surgical Oncology,* Vol.98. No.5, (October 2008), pp. 384–392, ISSN 0022-4790

Sexton, JA, (2008). Laparoscopic gastric resection for gastrointestinal stromal tumors. *Surgical Endoscopy,* Vol.22, No.12, (December 2008), pp.:2583–2587, ISSN 0930-2794

Shah, JN. (2005). Neoadjuvant therapy with imatinib mesylate for locally advanced GI stromal tumor. *Gastrointestinal Endoscopy,* Vol.61, No.4, (April 2005), pp. 625–627, ISSN 0016-5107

Shinomura, Y. (2005). Pathophysiology, diagnosis, and treatment of gastrointestinal stromal tumors. *Journal of Gastroenterology,* Vol.40, No.8, (August 2005), pp. 775-780, ISSN 0944-1174

Silberhumer, GR. (2009). Surgery for gastrointestinal stromal tumors of the stomach. *Journal of Gastrointestinal Surgery,* Vol.13, No.7, (July 2009), pp. 1213–1219, ISSN 1091-255X

Singer, S. (2002). Prognostic value of KIT mutation type, mitotic activity, and histologic subtype in gastrointestinal stromal tumors. *Journal of Clinical Oncology,* Vol.20, No.18, (September 2002), pp. 3898-3905, ISSN 0732-183X

Sjölund, K. (2010). Downsizing treatment with tyrosine kinase inhibitors in patients with advanced gastrointestinal stromal tumors improved resectability. *World Journal of Surgery,* Vol.34, No.9, (September 2010), pp. 2090-2097, ISSN 0364-2313 stromal tumours. *Nature,* Vol.467, No.7317, (October 2010), pp. 849-853, ISSN 0028-0836

Stroobants, S. (2003). ^{18}FDG-Positron emission tomography for the early prediction of response in advanced soft tissue sarcoma treated with imatinib mesylate (Glivec). *European Journal of Cancer,* Vol. 39, No. 14, (September 2003), pp. 2012-2020, ISSN 0959-8049

Van den Abbeele, AD. (2008). The lessons of GIST--PET and PET-CT- a new paradigm for imaging. *The Oncologist,* Vol.13m Suppl.2, (April 2008), pp. 8-13, ISSN 1083-7159

Verweij, J. (2004). Progression-free survival in gastrointestinal stromal tumours with high-dose imatinib: randomised trial. *Lancet,* Vol.364, No.9440, (October 2004), pp. 1127–1134, ISSN 0140-6736

West RB, Corless CL, Chen X et al (2004) The novel marker, DOG1, is expressed ubiquitously in gastrointestinal stromal tumors irrespective of KIT or PDGFRA mutation status. Am J Pathol 165(1):107–113

West, RB. (2004). The novel marker, DOG1, is expressed ubiquitously in gastrointestinal stromal tumors irrespective of KIT or PDGFRA mutation status. *American Journal of Pathology,* Vol.165, No.1, (July 2004), pp. 107-113, ISSN 0002-9440

Winer, JH. (2011). Management of recurrent gastrointestinal stromal tumors. *Journal of Surgical Oncology,* (February 2011), doi: 10.1002/jso.21890. [Epub ahead of print], ISSN 0022-4790

Woodall, CE, 3rd. (2009). An evaluation of 2537 gastrointestinal stromal tumors for a proposed clinical staging system. *Archives of Surgery,* Vol.144, No.7, (July 2009), pp. 670-678, ISSN 0004-0010

Yan, H. (2003). Prognostic assessment of gastrointestinal stromal tumor. *American Journal of Clinical Oncology,* Vol.26, No.3, (June 2003), pp. 221-228, ISSN 0277-3732

Yang, WL. (2009). Duodenal gastrointestinal stromal tumor: Clinical, pathologic, immunohistochemical characteristics, and surgical prognosis. *Journal of Surgical Oncology,* Vol.100, No.7, (December 2009), pp. 606–610, ISSN 0022-4790

Yoon, SS. (2007). Should surgical resection be combined with imatinib therapy for locally advanced or metastatic gastrointestinal stromal tumors? *Annals of Surgery Oncology,* Vol.14, No.6, (June 2007), pp. 1784-1786, ISSN 1068-9265

Zhu, J. (2010). A long-term follow-up of the imatinib mesylate treatment for the patients with recurrent GIST- the liver metastasis and the outcome.*BMC cancer,* Vol.13, No.10, (May 2010), pp. 199, ISSN 1471-2407

3

Molecularly Targeted Therapy: Imatinib and Beyond

Andrew Poklepovic and Prithviraj Bose
Massey Cancer Center, Division of Hematology, Oncology and Palliative Care
Virginia Commonwealth University, Richmond, Virginia,
USA

1. Introduction

This chapter will focus on the molecular biology of gastrointestinal stromal tumors, with a focus on therapy targeting the primary activating mutations in the KIT proto-oncogene. The studies that have led to the approval of imatinib and sunitinib will be reviewed. Additional novel agents under development will be discussed.

2. Background and histology

Gastrointestinal stromal tumors (GISTs) are rare tumors, with an estimated incidence of 1.5/100,000 persons per year (Nilsson, 2005). This number accounts for clinically relevant tumors, there is a much higher number of microscopic lesions that can be detected on pathologic specimens. The incidence of such microscopic subclinical lesions approaches 20% in surgical and autopsy specimens (Agaimy, 2007). GISTs account for the overwhelming majority of mesenchymal tumors arising in the GI tract. GISTs arise most frequently in the stomach (approximately 60%), and small bowel (30%), but these tumors can arise anywhere in the GI tract (DeiTos, 2011). GISTs are thought to originate from the interstitial cells of Cajal (GI pacemaker cells). These subepithelial neoplasms share a unique molecular and immunohistochemical signature. Morphologically, GISTs are subdivided into spindle cell, epithelioid cell, and mixed types, but these distinctions have little clinical relevance. Overt cytologic atypia and dedifferentiation are quite rare, and should lead to considerations of alternative diagnoses (DeiTos, 2011). Nearly all GISTs express immunoreactivity to c-KIT, also known as CD117 or stem cell growth factor receptor (SCFR). The KIT receptor is a membrane-bound class III receptor tyrosine kinase (RTK) encoded by the *KIT* proto-oncogene. This RTK is activated by the binding of mast cell growth factor (MGF), also known as stem cell factor. About 95% of GISTs overexpress KIT. DOG1 has also been used as a very sensitive and specific immunomarker. In a large pathology series, the overall sensitivity of DOG1 and KIT in GISTs was nearly identical: 94.4% and 94.7%, and results in GISTs were generally concordant. Gastric spindle cell GISTs were nearly uniformly positive for both markers, whereas DOG1 performed slightly better in gastric epithelioid GISTs that included a higher percentage of platelet derived growth factor receptor alpha (PDGFRA)-mutant GISTs. In the intestinal GISTs, KIT was slightly more sensitive than DOG1. Negativity for both DOG1 and KIT was observed in 2.6% of GISTs (Miettinen, 2009). In 80%

of cases, KIT overexpression is the result of activating mutations in exons 9, 11, 13 and 17 in the *KIT* proto-oncogene (Corless, 2008). Most *KIT* mutations (70%) affect exon 11 within the juxtamembrane domain, and result in constitutive activity of the RTK (Heinrich, 2008). Another clinically important mutation occurs in exon 9, part of the extracellular domain, and occurs almost exclusively in intestinal GIST (Ganjoo 2011). Over-expression without identifiable mutations also occurs, and the mechanism for over-expression of KIT in such cases is presently unclear. Approximately 5% of cases of GIST are immunohistochemically negative for KIT. Activating mutations in a related RTK, PDGFRA, account for most of these cases. KIT and *PDGFRA* mutations do appear to be mutually exclusive oncogenic mechanisms in GISTs. However, a small percentage of GISTs lack mutations in either RTK, and the molecular pathogenesis of these tumors remains unknown at this time. Although most GISTs are sporadic, familial cases with heritable mutations in the *KIT* gene have been identified. Rare syndromes include the Carney triad, which involves GIST, extra-adrenal paraganglionomas, and pulmonary chondromas. In the Carney-Stratakis syndrome, which is transmitted in an autosomal dominant fashion, only GISTs and the paraganglionomas are seen. There is also an increased risk of GIST in patients with neurofibromatosis type I (Kinoshita, 2004.) Pediatric GIST tumors are a distinctive subset, occur mostly in females, are *KIT/PDGFRA* wild-type, and generally follow an indolent course (Dei Tos, 2011).

3. Clinical presentation and staging

Common presentations of GISTs include an abdominal mass, pain or GI bleeding. Histologically, 70% are the spindle cell type, 20% the epithelioid type, and a mixed pattern is encountered in 10% of cases. Tumor size and mitotic rate are the most important determinants of aggressiveness, although location within the GI tract also matters. In general, intestinal GISTs are more aggressive than are gastric tumors. Indeed, there are different stage groupings for gastric, omental and small bowel, esophageal, colorectal and mesenteric primaries in the tumor-node-metastasis (TNM) system. A contrast-enhanced computed tomographic (CT) scan is generally the preferred initial imaging study for screening and staging, although magnetic resonance imaging (MRI), upper GI endoscopy, endoscopic ultrasound (EUS) and positron emission tomographic (PET) scanning using fluorodeoxyglucose (FDG) all have potential utility, depending on the clinical scenario. For example, EUS is the most accurate modality for distinguishing leiomyomas from other submucosal lesions. Preoperative biopsy is not generally recommended for a resectable lesion that is highly suspicious for GIST, unless metastatic disease is suspected, or neoadjuvant imatinib is being considered. Surgery remains the mainstay of local treatment of GIST. All localized GISTs ≥ 2 cm should be completely resected. There is no consensus on the management of smaller lesions. For potentially resectable GISTs, segmental (rather than peritumoral) visceral resection is preferred. Routine lymphadenectomy is unnecessary because nodal metastases are rare.

4. Targeting KIT in GIST

Imatinib mesylate is a competitive inhibitor of the Bcr-Abl, KIT and PDGFRA RTKs. The dramatic results of the IRIS (International Randomized Study of Interferon and STI571) trial in patients with chronic myelogenous leukemia (CML) revolutionized the treatment of that disease and ushered in a new era of molecularly targeted therapy in oncology (O'Brien, 2003). It subsequently became evident that imatinib induced dramatic, rapid and sustained clinical benefit in advanced GISTs as well. GISTs are exquisitely dependent on signaling via KIT or PDGFRA because of the activating mutations discussed above, a phenomenon termed "oncogene addiction". Molecularly targeted therapy with tyrosine kinase inhibitors (TKIs) such as imatinib or sunitinib blocks such signaling, and consequently also the downstream pathways. (**Figure 1**)

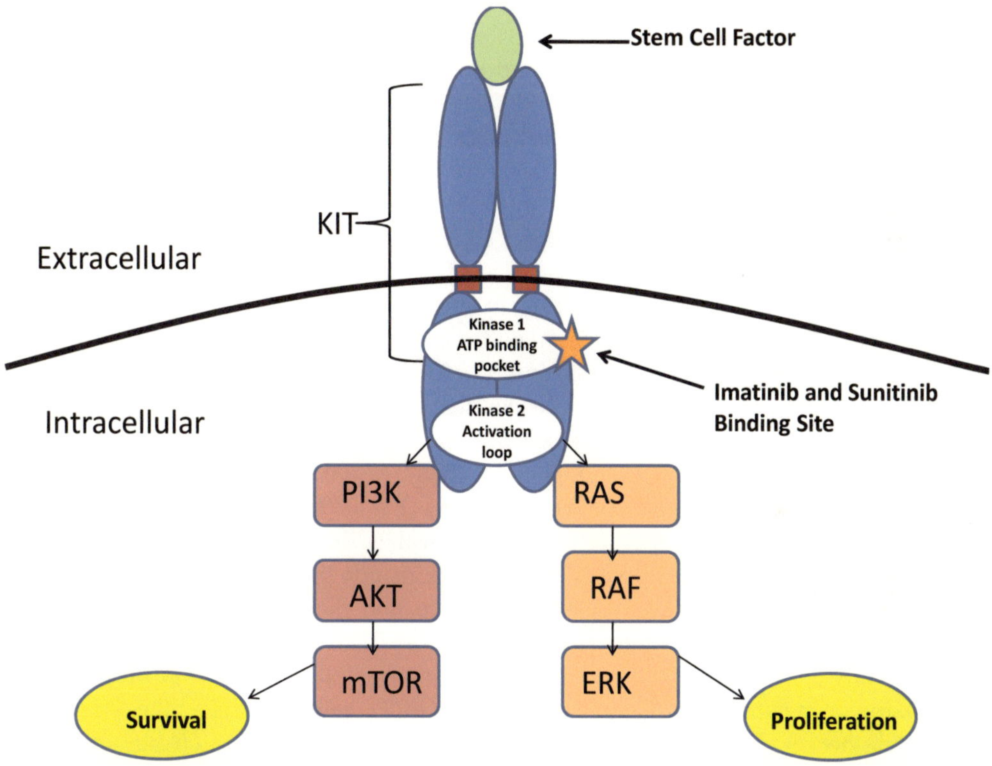

Fig. 1. A simplified schematic diagram of the KIT transmembrane receptor tyrosine kinase and downstream signaling pathways. Constitutive activation of KIT is caused by mutations in the extracellular domain (exon 9), the juxtamembrane domain (exon 11), or the intracytoplasmic kinase domain (exons 13 and 17) that result in different profiles of drug sensitivity/resistance. Activation of KIT leads to ERK activation, mTOR activation and JAK/STAT activation (not shown).

5. Characterization of response

An important consideration in the development of clinical trials in the modern era of targeted therapy is the measure of response. In 2000, a group of international experts agreed on standard criteria for measuring tumor response, called Response Evaluation Criteria in Solid Tumors (RECIST). Each lesion that is identified as a target lesion (>1 cm) is measured in one dimension, the longest diameter. A complete response (CR) is the disappearance of all target tumors. A partial response (PR) is a 30% or larger decrease in the sum of the longest diameters of the tumors. Progressive disease (PD) is a 20% or greater increase in the sum of the diameters. Stable disease (SD) refers to changes in tumor size that do not meet any of these criteria. RECIST has numerous shortcomings but remains the standard for evaluating response in clinical trials, although that is beginning to change. An increasing number of drugs in development inhibit tumor cell growth (cytostatic) and thus do not shrink the tumor, unlike conventional chemotherapeutic agents, which kill tumor cells (cytotoxic). Criticisms have been raised that tumor density or metabolic activity are not related to diameter, and clinically relevant responses are missed when using uni-dimensional measurements. To address this weakness, alternative criteria, including the Choi criteria, have been proposed. In GIST, tumors only rarely shrink greater than the 30% required for response characterization by RECIST, yet survival benefit of therapy is proven. Changes in tumor density rather than size appear to correlate better with response to these drugs, and prolonged disease stabilization rather than frank tumor shrinkage may be seen on imaging studies. Choi criteria use a 10 percent decrease in unidimensional tumor size or a 15 percent decrease in tumor density on contrast-enhanced CT scans (as reflected by differences in x-ray attenuation between a given material and water, expressed in Hounsfield units), to determine response. In one comparison study looking at RECIST criteria versus Choi criteria in 58 patients with GIST, responses by Choi criteria predicted disease-specific survival while RECIST criteria did not. Using RECIST, 28 (48%) patients showed response and 30 (52%) were nonresponders. Yet there was no statistically significant difference in time to progression between the two groups ($P = .2$). By the Choi criteria, however, 49 (84%) were good responders and 9 (16%) were not. The good responders had a longer time to progression than the poor responders ($P = .0002$). The Choi criteria also more accurately predicted disease-specific overall survival (OS) than did the RECIST criteria (Benjamin, 2007). Additional response criteria in use include the Southwest Oncology Group (SWOG) criteria, which monitors disease control rate, and characterizes anything that is not tumor growth as a response. Another approach is to evaluate metabolic activity using FDG-PET. In a study of 23 patients getting second line therapy with sunitinib after progression on imatinib, tumor metabolism was assessed with FDG-PET before and after the first 4 weeks of sunitinib therapy. Treatment response was expressed as the percent change in maximal standardized uptake value (SUV). The primary end point of time to tumor progression on the basis of RECIST criteria was compared with early PET results. Progression-free survival (PFS) was correlated with early FDG-PET metabolic response ($P < .0001$). Using -25% and +25% thresholds for SUV variations from baseline, early FDG-PET response was stratified into metabolic partial response, metabolically stable disease, or metabolically progressive disease; median PFS rates were 29, 16, and 4 weeks, respectively. Similarly, when a single FDG-PET result was considered after 4 weeks of sunitinib, the median PFS was 29 weeks for SUVs less than 8 g/mL versus 4 weeks for SUVs of 8 g/mL or greater ($P < .0001$). None of the patients with metabolically progressive disease subsequently responded according to RECIST criteria. Multivariate analysis showed shorter PFS in patients who had higher residual SUVs ($P < .0001$), primary resistance to imatinib ($P = .024$), or nongastric GIST ($P = .002$), regardless of the mutational status of the KIT and PDGFRA genes (Prior, 2009). To summarize, imaging evaluations of response to targeted therapy in GIST are evolving. It is important to keep in mind that tumor shrinkage alone may not correlate with response or survival in GIST in the context of the current arsenal of therapeutic agents.

6. Imatinib in the treatment of GIST

Imatinib is the standard of care for advanced, unresectable or metastatic GIST. It has improved median overall survival from 18 to 57 months, vastly changing the outlook for patients with this disease (Figure II). A single case was reported by Joensuu and colleagues showing a dramatic response to imatinib in a patient with metastatic GIST (Joensuu, 2001). This led to the subsequent treatment of 35 patients in a phase I study conducted by the European Organization for Research and Treatment for Cancer (EORTC), which showed a 54% PR and 37% SD rate (van Oosterom, 2002). In a subsequent large multicenter, randomized, open-label phase II study, patients with metastatic or unresectable GIST were treated with either imatinib 400 or 600 mg daily (Demetri, 2002). Patients whose tumors progressed on imatinib 400 mg were allowed to take the higher dose. Of the 147 patients treated, 53.7% had a PR and 27.9% had SD. Efficacy was based on the SWOG criteria and the median time to response was 13 weeks. The results of this trial led to Food and Drug Administration (FDA)-approval of imatinib for the treatment of unresectable or metastatic GIST in the United States (**Table 1**, page 6). Long-term follow-up analysis showed a 5-year OS rate of 57% in patients who responded to imatinib, and only a 9% 5-year OS rate in those who progressed. There also appears to be molecular heterogeneity in terms of survival on imatinib. Median OS was 63 months in patients with the more common c-KIT exon 11 mutation, compared with 44 months in patients with exon 9 mutations (Blanke 2008). This is also described in **Figure 2**, shown below.

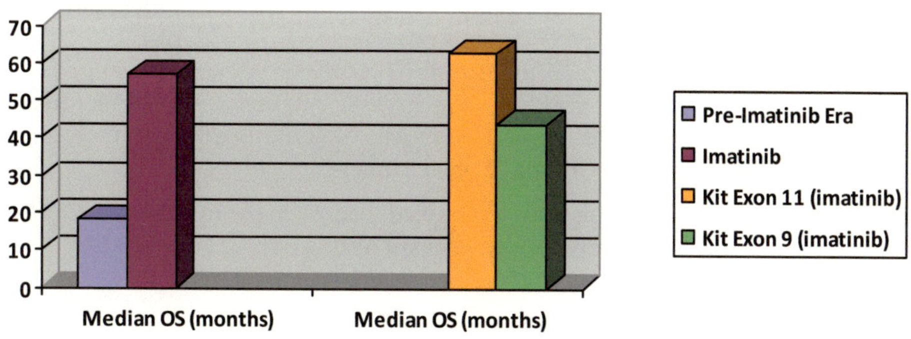

Fig. 2. Median overall survival in the pre-imatinib era compared to the long term survival data from the phase II study that led to the US FDA approval of imatinib in advanced GIST. Upon analysis of the long term survival data, it became clear that exon 9 mutations carry a worse prognosis than the more common exon 11 mutations (Blanke 2008) in imatinib-treated patients.

Registration trial	Treatment and comparison	Findings
Imatinib in unresectable or metastatic disease (Demetri GD, 2002)	400 mg or 600 mg imatinib p.o. daily in 147 patients. Comparison to historical controls SWOG criteria for response evaluation used, not RECIST	53.7% PR rate 27.9% SD rate 13.6% showed early resistance 0% CR rate Median PFS and OS identical on both arms Median survival 57 months for all patients 28% remained on therapy long-term Time to onset of response 3 months.
Sunitinib as second line therapy in patients intolerant/refractory to imatinib (Demetri GD, 2006)	Sunitinib 50 mg p.o. daily, for 4 weeks every 6 weeks. International study, 312 patients, randomized 2:1 in favor of sunitinib	27.3 weeks PFS on sunitinib; 6.4 weeks on placebo PR or SD for at least 6 months was observed for the three most common primary GIST genotypes: KIT exon 9 (58%), KIT exon 11 (34%), wild-type KIT/PDGFRA (56%) May have increased activity against exon 9 mutations.
Adjuvant imatinib after resection of GISTs ≥ 3 cm (DiMatteo, 2009)	Imatinib 400 mg p.o. daily for 1 year 713 patients randomized 1:1 to imatinib or placebo	Relapse free survival at 1 yr 98% with imatinib, and 83% with placebo

Abbreviations: CR, complete response, PR, partial response, SD, stable disease, PFS, progression-free survival, OS, overall survival, SWOG, Southwest Oncology Group, RECIST, Response Evaluation Criteria In Solid Tumors.

Table 1. Summary of the 3 major trials of targeted therapy in the treatment of GIST. Overview of treatment administered and relevant results.

7. Dose escalation of imatinib in advanced GIST

Like in CML, the use of higher doses of imatinib (800 mg vs 400 mg daily) upfront has not been found to be advantageous in terms of impacting overall survival, and 400 mg daily represents the standard initial dose for most patients. A meta-analysis performed in 2009 looked at two large randomized trials comparing two dosing regimens for advanced unresectable and metastatic GIST (MetaGIST, 2010). Two phase III studies (the EU-AUS and US-CDN studies) looked at standard dose imatinib (400mg once daily) and high dose imatinib (400mg twice daily). High dose therapy showed an initial improvement in progression free survival (PFS) at 2 years, which was no longer significant with long term followup. There are several possible contributing factors to this result. Nearly half of all patients in both studies had to have a dose reduction by 6 months, raising the question of long term tolerability. It is also possible that the PFS improvement at 2 years was due to dose-dependent mechanisms of resistance within the first 2 years, with alternate mechanisms affecting late resistance. The only identified predictive risk factor was the presence of *KIT* exon 9 mutations. For exon 9 mutations, there was a 42% reduction in the risk of progression or death in the high-dose group, compared to the low dose group. A non-significant 31% reduction in the risk of death was also seen. Exon 9 mutation rates remained low (8.1% in US-CDN and 15.6% in EU-AUS), and as such, true differences were difficult to detect even in the context of a meta-analysis. As such, there continues to be debate over the status of exon 9 mutations and initial choice of therapy, and there is disagreement amongst expert opinions and guidelines from the United States and Europe. Currently, the US National Comprehensive Cancer Network (NCCN) recommends that patients with documented exon 9 mutations in *KIT* be considered for dose escalation to 400mg twice daily, as tolerated. The European Society for Medical Oncology (ESMO) considers higher dose imatinib to be standard of care in this setting. Both recommend dose escalation to 400mg twice daily at the time of progression, regardless of mutation status. Stabilization of disease or even response can be seen after progression on standard doses of imatinib.

8. Pharmacokinetic considerations of therapy

Interpatient variability in pharmacokinetic exposure to the drug may also influence outcome. In this regard, monitoring of plasma levels of imatinib has been proposed, although its clinical impact remains unclear, pending further evaluation. In a pharmacokinetic study, clinical outcomes were correlated with imatinib trough levels at steady state. The median time to progression was 11.3 months for patients in the lowest C(min) quartile (Q1, < 1,110 ng/mL) compared with more than 30 months for those in the second through fourth quartiles (P = .0029) (Demetri, 2009). Prior surgery plays a substantial role in the bioavailability of TKI therapy, as all compounds currently used in the treatment of GIST are taken orally. Imatinib has an acid-dependent solubility, and plasma concentrations are significantly lower in patients who have undergone gastrectomy as part of prior GIST resection surgery (Yoo, 2010). Additionally, genetic polymorphisms affecting cellular uptake of imatinib have been shown to be important in CML patients. The intracellular uptake and retention of imatinib is dependent on the active transporter, organic cation transporter 1, (OCT-1). CML patients with low levels of OCT-1 required higher doses of imatinib to achieve response than patients with high levels of OCT-1 (White, 2007). This pharmacokinetic variability has not been explored in GISTs at this time, and testing of OCT-1 expression is not routine for these patients. Collectively, the evidence suggests that individualized tailoring of therapy to achieve optimal drug levels may play a role in the future.

9. Duration of therapy and side effect profile

For advanced disease, treatment with imatinib is indicated indefinitely: interruption of therapy leads to rapid disease progression in most patients, even after years of responsive or stable disease (Le Cesne, 2010b). Common side effects (>20%) of imatinib include fluid retention, fatigue, abdominal pain, skin rash, muscle cramps, nausea, vomiting, and diarrhea (Dagher, 2002). Edema is generally superficial and confined to the eyelids and extremities, but pleural effusion and ascites can be seen. Macrocytosis is frequently seen, as is a mild anemia with chronic use or at higher doses. Neutropenia, hypophosphatemia, gynecomastia, lung, liver and cardiac toxicity are occasionally reported, and rarely, tumor lysis syndrome may occur. Depression has been noted, and has rarely required discontinuation of the drug. Intratumoral hemorrhage of large tumors has been seen in responding patients, and hemoglobin should be monitored for patients with bulky disease as they start therapy.

10. Sunitinib as second line therapy

Sunitinib is another multitargeted TKI, inhibiting KIT, PDGFRA, PDGFRB, FLT3, vascular endothelial growth factor receptors (VEGFR) 1,2 and 3, RET and colony stimulating factor-1R (CSF-1R) tyrosine kinases. Sunitinib represents the standard of care in advanced renal cell carcinoma. Sunitinib is approved in the US at a dose of 50 mg daily for four out of every six weeks for imatinib-refractory or –intolerant advanced GISTs . This approval was based on an increasing number of reports indicating efficacy of sunitinib in these settings, which culminated in a large international phase III placebo-controlled trial. In this trial, 312 patients were randomized in a 2:1 ratio to receive sunitinib (n=207) or placebo (n=105) in a blinded fashion. Study medication was given orally once daily at a 50-mg starting dose in 6-week cycles with 4 weeks on and 2 weeks off treatment. The primary endpoint was time to tumor progression. The trial was unblinded early when a planned interim analysis showed significantly longer time to tumor progression in the sunitinib arm. Median time to tumor progression was 27.3 weeks (95% CI 16.0–32.1) in patients receiving sunitinib and 6.4 weeks (4.4–10.0) in those on placebo (hazard ratio 0.33; $p<0.0001$) (Demetri, 2006). The results of this pivotal study are also reviewed in table 1. While the approved dose of sunitinib for GIST in the United States is 50mg daily for 4 weeks followed by 2 weeks rest, continuous dosing at 37.5 mg daily appears to be similarly safe and effective (George, 2005). Common side effects of sunitinib include fatigue, diarrhea, anorexia, nausea, vomiting, abdominal pain, myelosuppression, hypothyroidism, and discoloration of skin and hair. Hypertension, cardiac and renal toxicity, elevations in serum amylase and lipase, and palmar-plantar erythrodysesthesia are less commonly seen. There may be a selective benefit to sunitinib versus imatinib, depending on the site of the *KIT* mutation. GISTs with the more common exon 11 *KIT* mutations are more sensitive to imatinib than exon 9 mutants. Conversely, sunitinib appears to benefit those with exon 9 mutations significantly more than those with exon 11 mutations. This was shown in a recent phase I/II study of patients who were resistant/intolerant to imatinib. Clinical benefit (PR or SD for at least 6 months) with sunitinib was observed for the three most common primary GIST genotypes: *KIT* exon 9 (58%), *KIT* exon 11 (34%), and wild-type *KIT/PDGFRA* (56%). Progression-free survival (PFS) was significantly longer for patients with primary *KIT* exon 9 mutations ($P = 0.0005$) or with a wild-type genotype ($P = 0.0356$) than for those with *KIT* exon 11 mutations (Heinrich, 2008). One confounder regarding sunitinib and exon 11 is that all published studies to date have evaluated sunitinib in the second line setting, after imatinib failure. It is known that secondary mutations will confer resistance to imatinib, and may appear years after imatinib therapy. These mutations are nonrandom and cluster in exons 13 and 14, part of the drug binding pocket of the receptor, as well as in exon 17, which encodes the kinase activation loop. Secondary kinase mutations were significantly more common in GISTs with primary *KIT* exon 11 mutations than in those with exon 9 mutations (73% *v* 19%; P = 0.0003) (Heinrich, 2008). It is not known if sunitinib will have the same efficacy profile in therapy-naïve patients with GIST.

11. Adjuvant therapy

As in other malignancies, the success of imatinib in the setting of advanced disease led to its study in the adjuvant and neoadjuvant settings. After a phase II trial (ACOSOG Z9000) of one year of adjuvant imatinib in patients with high-risk completely resected GIST yielded encouraging findings, the pivotal phase III ACOSOG Z9001 trial was conducted. This trial, which was stopped early because of significantly fewer recurrences in the treatment arm, led to the approval in the US of adjuvant imatinib (400 mg daily) for patients with resected GISTs ≥ 3 cm in size, without indicating the optimal duration of therapy. 359 patients were randomized to imatinib and 354 to placebo. In this trial, imatinib significantly prolonged relapse free survival (RFS) compared with placebo (98% vs. 83% at 1 year; overall hazard ratio 0.35; one-sided P < 0.0001) (**Table I**, DiMatteo, 2009). Similar large phase III trials have been conducted in Europe, one with overall survival as the primary endpoint. Crucial to determining the need for, or optimal duration of, adjuvant imatinib is accurate risk-stratification, and ESMO guidelines state that adjuvant imatinib can be "proposed as an option" for patients at substantial risk for relapse, calling for shared decision-making in situations of uncertainty. An additional study of 105 patients in China looked at 3 years of adjuvant imatinib 400mg daily versus observation in patients with resected high-risk or intermediate-risk GIST. This duration of adjuvant imatinib treatment is 2 years longer than the published ACOSOG Z9001 study. Relapse free survival (RFS) at 1, 2 and 3 years was higher in the treatment group than in the control group (100% vs. 90% at 1 year; 96% vs. 57% at 2 years; 89% versus 48% at 3 years; P < 0.001, HR = .188). Subgroup analyses showed that adjuvant therapy significantly decreased the risk of recurrence in patients, whether at high risk or at intermediate risk, compared with control patients (3-year RFS 95% vs. 72% in intermediate risk; 85% versus 31% in high risk, P < 0.001). In addition, adjuvant imatinib treatment decreased the risk of death (P = .039, HR = .254) (Li, 2011). Apart from the risk factors mentioned above, tumor rupture and incomplete resection are independent risk factors that negatively impact disease-free survival.

12. Neoadjuvant therapy

Since surgery is the only potentially curative option for GIST, neoadjuvant imatinib has been investigated in an effort to improve surgical outcomes. At this time, there are no randomized clinical trials from which to draw conclusions. Data from several case reports, retrospective series and one phase II trial suggest a role for neoadjuvant imatinib. The RTOG 0132/ACRIN 6665 trial was a prospective phase II study evaluating safety and efficacy of neoadjuvant imatinib (600 mg/day) for patients with primary GIST or the pre-operative use of imatinib in patients with operable metastatic GIST. The trial continued post-operative imatinib for 2 years. Sixty-three patients were entered (52 analyzable), 30 patients with primary GIST (Group A) and 22 with recurrent, metastatic GIST (Group B). Responses (RECIST) in Group A were: 7% partial, 83% stable, 10% unknown, and in Group B were: 4.5% partial, 91% stable, 4.5% progression. Two-year progression-free survival was

83% in Group A, and 77% in Group B. Estimated 2-year overall survival in Group A was 93%, and 91% in Group B. Complications of surgery and imatinib toxicity were minimal (Eisenberg BL, 2009). One criticism of this study is that the duration of preoperative imatinib was relatively short (8-12 weeks), which is likely too soon for response to fully manifest. Long term followup of the original study using imatinib in advanced or metastatic disease showed that in 25% of the patients, an objective response was achieved only after 5.3 to 39 months of imatinib treatment (Blanke, 2008). While CT scans remain the standard imaging modality for assessment of response in this setting, PET scans may be helpful when an expeditious assessment of response is needed. In general, neoadjuvant imatinib is indicated for patients with marginally resectable tumors and for those who have potentially resectable disease but with the risk of significant surgical morbidity. Some advocate its use only in the context of clinical trials, and others reserve it for high-risk patients. A dose of 400 mg daily is most commonly used, although 800 mg/day is reasonable for patients with exon 9 mutations. Sunitinib is also being evaluated in the neoadjuvant setting in a current clinical trial. The duration of therapy varies from 3 to 12 months, and periodic imaging evaluations are needed. The optimal duration of neoadjuvant imatinib and timing of surgery (at first resectability versus once the response has reached a plateau) have to be individualized. For responding patients, at least a year of adjuvant imatinib after resection is recommended, with longer durations being considered by many. Additionally, imatinib has been used pre- and post-operatively with resection in patients with liver metastases. In one study, forty one patients with liver metastases were randomized to imatinib plus resection (6 months neoadjuvant imatinib, then resection, followed by adjuvant imatinib), versus imatinib alone. In the 36-month followup period, the combination group had 1- and 3-year survival rates of 100% and 89.5%, while the imatinib-only group had survival rates of 85% and 60% respectively (P = 0.03) (Xia, 2010) In the absence of clear randomized data, coupled with the long term tolerability of imatinib, it seems reasonable to pursue neoadjuvant and adjuvant imatinib in patients that are at high risk for surgical complications, or unresectable at presentation. Enrollment onto neoadjuvant clinical trials will be imperative to determining the optimum timing, duration, and response to neoadjuvant therapy.

13. Molecular considerations to targeted therapy

Agents within the same class of targeted therapies may have different properties that appear to play a role in response and side effect profiles. Even closely related compounds interact with their binding sites differently, and bind with different affinities to other RTKs. Imatinib works by competitively and reversibly binding to the ATP-binding pocket of KIT, resulting in stabilization of the inactive conformation of the kinase domain (Gajiwala, 2009). This specificity for the inactive conformation of KIT helps explain why certain mutations, such as the exon 17 activation loop (A-loop) mutation confer resistance to imatinib (Demetri GD, 2011). Additionally, mutations in the ATP pocket, such as exon 13 and 14 mutations lead to imatinib resistance. Sunitinib is a smaller molecule than imatinib, and mutations in the binding pocket do not confer the same resistance as they do with imatinib. The differences in binding properties enable sunitinib to overcome some, but not all, secondary mutations that arise on imatinib therapy. As sunitinib also binds to the ATP-binding pocket with affinity for the inactive conformation of the enzyme, mutations in the A-loop also confer drug resistance to sunitinib (Demetri GD, 2011). Dasatnib is another molecule with binding affinity towards KIT. Its chemical structure is different from imatinib and sunitinib in that it is able to bind to the ATP-binding pocket regardless of the conformation of the kinase activation loop (Schittenhelm, 2006). Dasatinib is being studied in GIST in ongoing clinical trials. Molecular characterization of primary and secondary *KIT* mutations appear below in **Figure 3**.

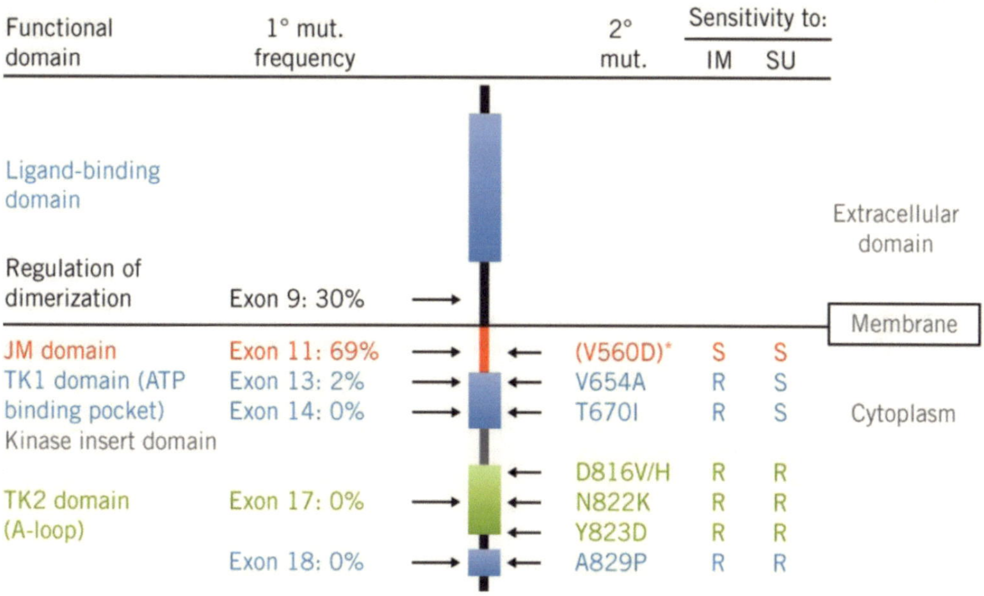

Fig. 3. Overview of the KIT protein, showing functional domains, and location of primary (1) and secondary (2) mutations (mut.) Frequencies of primary KIT mutations, specific secondary mutations, and resistance (R) or sensitivity (S) to imatinib (IM) or sunitinib (S) are as reported in the phase I/II trial of sunitinib in advanced GIST after imatinib failure (Heinrich, 2008). Reproduced, with permission, from Gajiwala, 2009. © 2009, National Academy of Sciences, USA.

14. New therapies in development

Several compounds are being investigated clinically in advanced GIST, as frontline therapy or after imatinib failure. In general, these compounds are directed at the RTKs KIT and PDGFRA. Oral masitinib was evaluated in 30 imatinib-naïve patients with advanced GIST (Le Cesne, 2010a) Masitinib has greater in-vitro activity and selectivity for the wild-type c-KIT receptor and the juxtamembrane domain mutation (exon 11) than imatinib. In a phase II study, the response rate (RR) at 2 months was 20% according to RECIST and 86% according to FDG-PET response criteria. Best responses were a CR in 1 of 30 patients, PR in 15 of 30 patients, SD in 13 of 30 patients, and PD occurred in 1 of 30 patients (disease control rate 96.7%). The OS rate at 2 and 3 years was high at 89.9%. There are plans to take masitinib forward in a phase III trial. Nilotinib is a second generation BCR/ABL TKI that is approved in the US for use in CML, both upfront and in patients resistant or intolerant to imatinib. Nilotinib has improved cellular uptake when compared to imatinib, and has been shown to have some preliminary activity in GIST in phase II studies. Thirty-five patients with intolerance or resistance to both imatinib and sunitinib were enrolled and treated with nilotinib 400 mg twice daily. Disease control rate (CR+PR+SD) at week 24 was 29% (90% confidence interval, 16.4%-43.6%) (Sawaki, 2011). The median PFS was 113 days, and the median OS was 310 days. Nilotinib is entering a pivotal multicenter phase III study versus imatinib in front line therapy. Vatalanib (PTK787/ZK 222584) is another oral TKI that inhibits KIT, PDGFRs and VEGFRs. Forty-five patients whose metastatic GIST had progressed on imatinib were enrolled. Nineteen (42.2%) patients had also received prior sunitinib. Vatalanib 1250 mg was administered orally daily. Eighteen patients (40.0%) had clinical benefit including 2 confirmed PRs (duration, 9.6 and 39.4 months) and 16 (35.6%) with stable disease, median duration 12.5 months (Joensuu, 2011). Everolimus is a member of the class of compounds known as mammalian target of rapamycin (mTOR) inhibitors. The protein mTOR is part of the phosphatidyl-inositol-3-kinase (PI3K) pathway, activated downstream of KIT. Everolimus is being investigated in combination therapy with imatinib. A phase I/II study of the addition of everolimus to 600mg imatinib daily in patients with progressive disease showed the combination to be tolerable and safe, and efficacy data met the predetermined endpoint for further study (Schoffski, 2010). Finally, some PDGFRA mutations such as D842V confer relative resistance to imatinib. There is no known effective treatment for these PDGFRA-mutant tumors, but studies using crenolanib, a potent PDGFR inhibitor with preclinical activity against D842V and other PDGFRA mutants, are underway.

15. Conclusion

Understanding the molecular biology of genetic mutations in GISTs has dramatically altered the landscape of therapy. It has been transformed from a disease for which no therapies were effective and lifespan of patients with advanced disease was invariably short, to a disease in which there are effective therapies promising prolonged survival with tolerable side effects. There are over 10 rationally targeted agents in clinical trials at the time of this publication, targeting primary mutations, accessory pathways, as well as specific resistance mutations. As we acquire a deeper understanding of the primary and secondary mutations, oncologists may one day be able to profile an individual patient's GIST mutations, and select drug therapy based on optimum activity against that specific mutation. At the time of progression, the mutations can be re-characterized and the next line of therapy selected based on the new mutational status. Hopefully, in the not too distant future, GIST, like chronic phase CML, will end up becoming a disease where the vast majority of patients can expect to lead normal lives with minimal side effects from their daily oral treatment.

16. References

Agaimy et al. Minute gastric sclerosing stromal tumors (GIST tumorlets) are common in adults and frequently show c-KIT mutations. Am J Surg Pathol 2007;3:113-20.

Benjamin et al. We should desist using RECIST, at least in GIST. J Clin Oncol. 2007 May 1;25(13):1760-4.

Blanke CD et al. Long term results from a randomized phase II trial of standard-dose versus higher-dose imatinib mesylate for patients with unresectable or metastatic gastrointestinal stromal tumors expressing KIT. J Clin Oncol 2008, Feb;26 (4):620-5

Corless CL, Heinrich MC. Molecular pathobiology of gastrointestinal stromal sarcomas. *Annu Rev Pathol* 2008;3:557-86.

Dagher R, et al. Approval summary: imatinib mesylate in the treatment of metastatic and/or unresectable malignant gastrointestinal stromal tumors. Clin Cancer Res 2002, Oct; 8:3034

Dei Tos, et al. Gastrointestinal stromal tumors: The histology report Digestive and liver disease, 43S (2011) S304-309

Demetri GD, et al. Efficacy and safety of imatinib mesylate in advanced gastrointestinal stromal tumors. N Engl J Med 2002 Aug; 347: 472-80

Demetri GD et al. Efficacy and safety of sunitinib in patients with advanced gastrointestinal stromal tumour after failure of imatinib: a randomised controlled trial. Lancet. 2006 Oct 14;368(9544):1329-38.

Demetri GD et al. Imatinib plasma levels are correlated with clinical benefit in patients with unresectable/metastatic gastrointestinal stromal tumors. J Clin Oncol. 2009 Jul 1;27(19):3141-7.

Demetri GD. Differential protperties of current tyrosine kinase inhibitors in gastrointestinal stromal tumors. Seminars in oncology, 2011 Apr; 38 (2) suppl 1: s10-s19

DiMatteo RP et al. Placebo-Controlled Randomized Trial of Adjuvant Imatinib Mesylate Following the Resection of Localized, Primary Gastrointestinal Stromal Tumor (GIST). Lancet. 2009 March 28; 373(9669): 1097–1104.

Eisenberg BL, Phase II trial of neoadjuvant/adjuvant imatinib mesylate (IM) for advanced primary and metastatic/recurrent operable gastrointestinal stromal tumor (GIST): early results of RTOG 0132/ACRIN 6665. J Surg Oncol. 2009;99(1):42.

Ganjoo KN et al. Current and emerging pharmacological treatments for gastrointestinal stromal tumor. Drugs. 2011 Feb 12;71(3):321-30.

George S et al. Clinical evaluation of continuous daily dosing of sunitinib malate in patients with advanced gastrointestinal stromal tumour after imatinib failure. Eur J Cancer. 2009 Jul;45(11):1959-68

Gajiwala KS et al. KIT kinase mutants show unique mechanisms of drug resistance to imatinib and sunitinib in gastrointestinal stromal tumor patients. Proc Natl Acad Scie USA 2009; 106:1542-7

Heinrich MC et al Primary and Secondary Kinase Genotypes Correlate With the Biological and Clinical Activity of Sunitinib in Imatinib-Resistant Gastrointestinal Stromal Tumor. Jour Clin Oncol 2008 Nov; 26 (33): 5352-59

Joensuu H, Roberts PJ, Sarlomo-Rikala M, et al. Effect of the tyrosine kinase inhibitor STI571 in a patient with a metastatic gastrointestinal stromal tumor. N Engl J Med 2001 Apr; 344 (14): 1052-6

Joensuu H et al. Vatalanib for metastatic gastrointestinal stromal tumour (GIST) resistant to imatinib: final results of a phase II study. Br J Cancer. 2011 May 24;104(11):1686-90

Kinoshita et al. Absence of c-kit gene mutations in gastrointestinal stromal tumors from neurofibromatosis type 1 patients. J Pathol 2004; 202:80-5.

Le Cesne A et al. Phase II study of oral masitinib mesilate in imatinib-naïve patients with locally advanced or metastatic gastro-intestinal stromal tumour (GIST). Eur J Cancer. 2010 May;46(8):1344-51

Le Cesne A et al. Discontinuation of imatinib in patients with advanced gastrointestinal stromal tumours after 3 years of treatment: an open-label multicentre randomised phase 3 trial. Lancet Oncol. 2010 Oct;11(10):942-9

Li J et al. Post-operative imatinib in patients with intermediate or high risk gastrointestinal stromal tumor. Eur J Surg Oncol. 2011 Apr;37(4):319-24.

MetaGIST. Comparison of two doses of imatinib for the treatment of unresectable or metastatic gastrointestinal stromal tumors: a meta-analysis of 1.640 patients. J Clin Oncol, Mar 2010, 1247-53

Miettinen M et al. DOG1 antibody in the differential diagnosis of gastrointestinal stromal tumors: a study of 1840 cases. Am J Surg Pathol. 2009 Sep;33(9):1401-8.

Nilsson et al. Gastrointestinal stromal tumors: incidence, prevalence, clinical course, and prognostication in the pre-imatinib era-a population based study in western Sweden. Cancer, 2005;103:821-9.

O'Brien, et al. Imatinib compared with interferon and low-dose cytarabine for newly diagnosed chronic-phase chronic myeloid leukemia. N Engl J Med. 2003 Mar 13;348(11):994-1004.

Prior et al. Early prediction of response to sunitinib after imatinib failure by 18F-fluorodeoxyglucose positron emission tomography in patients with gastrointestinal stromal tumor. J Clin Oncol. 2009 Jan 20;27(3):439-45

Sawaki A et al. Phase 2 study of nilotinib as third-line therapy for patients with gastrointestinal stromal tumor. Cancer. 2011 Mar 31

Schittenhelm MM et al. Dasatinib (BMS-365825), a dual SCR/ABL kinase inhibitor, inhibits the kinase activity of wild-type, juxtamembrane, and activation loop mutant KIT isoforms associated with human malignancies. Cancer Res, 2006 Jan 1; 66(1):473-81

Schoffski P et al. A phase I-II study of everolimus (RAD001) in combination with imatinib in patients with imatinib-resistant gastrointestinal stromal tumors. Ann Oncol. 2010 Oct;21(10):1990-8

van Oosterom AT, et al. Update of phase I study of imatinib (STI571) in advanced soft tissue sarcomas and gastrointestinal stromal tumors: a report of the EORTC Soft Tissue and Bone Sarcoma Group. Eur J Cancer 2002 Sep; 38 Suppl. 5: S83-7

White et al. Most CML patients who have a suboptimal response to imatinib have low OCT-1 activity: higher doses of imatinib may overcome the negative impact of low OCT-1 activity. Blood. 2007 Dec 1;110(12):4064-72.

Xia L et al. Resection combined with imatinib therapy for liver metastases of gastrointestinal stromal tumors. Surg Today. 2010 Oct;40(10):936-42

Yoo C, Ryu MH, Kang BW et al (2010) Cross-Sectional study of imatinib plasma trough levels in patients with advanced gastrointestinal stromal tumors: impact of gastrointestinal resection on exposure to imatinib. J Clin Oncol 556:43–46

4

Surgical Treatment of Gastrointestinal Stromal Tumors (GISTs)

António M. Gouveia[1,3,4] and José Manuel Lopes[2,3,4]
[1]*Department of Surgery, Hospital de São João, Porto,*
[2]*Department of Pathology, Hospital de São João, Porto,*
[3]*Faculdade de Medicina do Porto,*
[4]*IPATIMUP,*
Portugal

1. Introduction

Gastrointestinal stromal tumors (GISTs) are the most common gastrointestinal tract (GI) mesenchymal tumors (Mazur and Clark 1983; Howe, Karnell et al. 2001), accounting for ~1-3% of all malignant neoplasms in this location. Most GISTs are sporadic, but there are hereditary forms, including some families with germline *KIT* and *PDGFRA* gene mutations. GIST diagnosis must be confirmed by immunohistochemistry of tumors, and integrated with other clinical and morphological features. GISTs usually express CD117 (95%) and CD34 (70%). Biological behavior is uncertain and classification (including largest size, mitotic rate and GI site) in risk categories is useful for predicting clinical behavior of GISTs. Other parameters have been described as prognostic of GISTs, including RKIP expression (Martinho, Gouveia et al. 2009). These tumors are characterized by oncogene mutations in *KIT* (up to ~85%) or *PDGFRA* (5-8%) receptor tyrosine kinases (RTKs) genes (Heinrich, Corless et al. 2003; Corless and Heinrich 2008; Gomes, Gouveia et al. 2008; Hoeben, Schoffski et al. 2008; Gajiwala, Wu et al. 2009; Liegl-Atzwanger, Fletcher et al. 2010), and rarely BRAF (Agaram, Wong et al. 2008; Agaimy, Terracciano et al. 2009; Martinho, Gouveia et al. 2009; Hostein, Faur et al. 2010); 10-15% does not harbor any of the aforementioned gene mutations: so called wild-type GISTs. *KIT/ PDGFR* mutations in GISTs are biodiversity markers, tyrosine kinase inhibitor (TKI) targets, predictive markers of TKI response, prognostic markers of tumor recurrence/progression, and frequent cause of TKI resistance. Thus, good clinical practice in bio-therapeutic decision of GIST patients should include mutational analysis status of the tumors.
Most importantly, complete surgical resection, without lymph node dissection, is considered standard treatment for primary localized GISTs (without peritoneal dissemination or metastatic disease), and is the only potential curative treatment for patients harboring these tumors.

2. Localized primary disease

There is a general consensus that the definitive treatment of primary GISTs with dimensions ≥ 2 cm and without evidence of peritoneal dissemination or distant metastases is complete macroscopic surgical resection (Casali and Blay 2010; Demetri, von Mehren et al. 2010). However, when esophagogastric or duodenal subepithelial nodules with < 2 cm diameter are detected, the standard procedure consists in endoscopic ultrasound (EUS) assessment and active surveillance of the individual patient, because many of these small nodules, when they correspond to GISTs, are tumors of low biological risk (Fletcher, Berman et al. 2002; Miettinen and Lasota 2006) or whose clinical behavior remains to be clarified. Surgery is reserved for patients whose tumor increases in dimension or is symptomatic. The results of a recent retrospective analysis (Lok, Lai et al. 2009) indicate that only some (3 out of 23; 13.0%) of the small tumors without high-risk EUS characteristics (large dimension, irregular extraluminal limits, heterogeneous echo pattern, presence of cystic areas, and hyperechoic foci) progressed during the long-term follow-up with EUS. As an alternative, the decision can be shared in an individual base with the patient, either to opt for an initial histological evaluation (needle biopsy) or for the tumor excision, when the morbidity is not substantial. On the other hand, when facing intra-abdominal nodules without endoscopic evaluation, the laparoscopy/laparotomy resection is the standard approach. Also for rectal nodules (or in the recto-vaginal space), the best management must be the accomplishment of biopsy/resection, after EUS evaluation, regardless of the tumor dimension, because GISTs in this location display high biological risk, and the local implications of a surgical intervention in this region is more critical, mostly in tumors of great dimensions.

The guidelines of the ESMO and the NCCN coincide in the recommendation that tumors with dimension > 2 cm must be resected (Casali and Blay 2010; Demetri, von Mehren et al. 2010), because being GISTs, they imply a higher risk of aggressive behavior.

For patients with localized primary GIST, the surgical resection continues to be the only possibility of cure of their illness. In our experience we obtained complete macroscopic resection (R0 or R1) in 92.3% of GISTs and microscopic negative margins (R0) in 75% of cases. 5-year disease-specific survival (DSS) and recurrence-free survival (RFS) was 87.7% and 89.8%, respectively, after surgical resection of patient's primary GIST. The recurrence rate was significantly ($p=0.045$) lower in R0 cases. In the multivariate analysis, only the presence of macroscopic residual tumor (R2) was significantly associated ($p=0.013$) with shorter DSS (Gouveia, Pimenta et al. 2008). The DSS and RFS values in our patients fit with results published in other studies (DeMatteo, Lewis et al. 2000; Crosby, Catton et al. 2001; Fujimoto, Nakanishi et al. 2003; Langer, Gunawan et al. 2003; Lin, Huang et al. 2003; Wong, Young et al. 2003; Bucher, Taylor et al. 2004; Bucher, Egger et al. 2006; Bumming, Ahlman et al. 2006). The recurrence rate was significantly lower in R0 cases, but in multivariate analysis only R2 resection was significantly associated with shorter survival of patients. According to the actual consensus recommendations (Casali and Blay 2010; Demetri, von Mehren et al. 2010), our results underline the prognostic importance of complete macroscopic surgical tumor resection, with the aim of achieving negative microscopic margins, and avoiding tumor rupture.

The surgery of GISTs should allow a complete margin of normal tissue around the primary tumor. The revision of most important published series shows that several authors refer to complete macroscopic resection (Ng, Pollock et al. 1992; Crosby, Catton et al. 2001; Pierie, Choudry et al. 2001; Eisenberg and Judson 2004; Boni, Benevento et al. 2005; Wu, Lee et al. 2006) of the tumors, whereas others specify R0 resection (Connolly, Gaffney et al. 2003; Langer, Gunawan et al. 2003; Wu, Langerman et al. 2003; Aparicio, Boige et al. 2004; Heinrich and Corless 2005; Bucher, Egger et al. 2006; Wardelmann, Buttner et al. 2007) as the standard procedure for the surgical treatment of GISTs. Some authors sustain that the microscopic status of the surgical margins (positive or negative), in contrast to the results obtained with other malignant solid tumors, does not influences the survival of patients, or even the recurrence of GISTs (DeMatteo, Lewis et al. 2000; Pierie, Choudry et al. 2001; Demetri, Baker et al. 2007). In a study of 200 patients with GIST, DeMatteo *et al.* (DeMatteo, Lewis et al. 2000) report that the microscopic margins do not significantly influence the evolution of the tumors and that recurrence occur most probably due to the intrinsic characteristics of the tumors. However, in the reported series, the relative small number of cases with positive microscopic margins after macroscopically complete resection is an important limitation to the clarification of the aforementioned author's suggestion. Additionally, this series included a substantial number of large dimension GISTs with high biological risk, in which complete macroscopic resection may not prevent the occurrence of recurrence (e.g., metastases) of the tumor or the shorter survival of these patients. In fact, the analysis of the results reported by DeMatteo *et al.* confirms that most resections were performed in patients with large GISTs with high biological risk (Lin, Huang et al. 2003; Bucher, Egger et al. 2006). The value of negative surgical margin, for instance in GISTs > 10 cm, is highly controversial, since it is possible to argue that those tumors may release to the peritoneal cavity cells not detectable clinically (DeMatteo, Lewis et al. 2000; Crosby, Catton et al. 2001). In addition, some of these reported results may be biased by the effect of adjuvant treatment performed in advanced or incompletely removed GISTs (He, Wang et al. 1988; DeMatteo, Lewis et al. 2000).

Other authors suggest that R0 resections may influence the prognosis of patients (Lehnert 1998; Pidhorecky, Cheney et al. 2000; Langer, Gunawan et al. 2003; Lin, Huang et al. 2003; Wu, Langerman et al. 2003; Yan, Marchettini et al. 2003; Bucher, Egger et al. 2006; Bumming, Ahlman et al. 2006; Hinz, Pauser et al. 2006; Ahmed, Welch et al. 2008); however, these results can also be influenced by the number of incomplete resections in GISTs of high biological risk (Lin, Huang et al. 2003).

Similar to the reports of DeMatteo *et al.* e Pierie *et al.* (Pierie, Choudry et al. 2001), our own results reinforce that complete macroscopic resection of GISTs has a positive impact in the prognosis, being significantly shorter the specific survival of patients with R2 tumor margin status.

Despite the remaining controversy, R1 margins resection may expose patients to a higher risk of tumoral locoregional recurrence of GISTs.

ESMO and NCCN recommend that in cases with R1 resections one should consider widening of resection, whenever the exact location of the lesion is possible to identify and the risk of surgical morbidity is low.

The surgical management recommended for small intestinal GISTs is segmental resection with 2-3 cm, and for gastric GISTs 1-2 cm free macroscopically margins (Dematteo, Heinrich et al. 2002; Matthews, Walsh et al. 2002; Wardelmann, Buttner et al. 2007; Hohenberger and Eisenberg 2010). An intraoperative histological frozen examination of peri-tumoral tissues must be compulsory whenever there is a possibility of not avoiding positive tumor surgical margins.

Usually, the resection causes low morbidity in tumors <10 cm, localized to stomach or small intestine. In contrast to more common gastrointestinal (GI) carcinomas, GIST does not originate from the epithelial layers of GI tract and, therefore, they present different biology and behavior implications. These facts are important for the surgical margins status procedures and locoregional lymph node management. The surgical procedures can differ, depending on the organ where GIST originates, on its precise localization, and the dimensions of the tumor. The treatment goal is complete resection of GIST, with negative microscopic margins (R0) and preservation of an intact pseudocapsule (i.e. preventing the tumoral rupture) (Casali and Blay 2010; Demetri, von Mehren et al. 2010).

As GIST does not have generally intraparietal infiltrative features, the attainment of wide surgical margins rarely associates with a prognostic benefit for the patients. The present recommendations for surgical margins are based on expert experience, consensus meeting reports, and application of the pathobiology concepts on GIST (Casali and Blay 2010; Demetri, von Mehren et al. 2010). In fact, there is no prospective conclusive evidence that allows predicting the relation between the extension of resection margins and the risk of local or distant recurrence of GISTs.

The wedge resection is the most frequent option for GISTs located in the stomach and the segmental resection is the procedure of choice for small bowel tumors. For GISTs of large dimensions in gastric lesser curvature and/or with pyloric involvement, wedge resection may not be possible, and a distal gastrectomy might be a more adequate procedure. Total gastrectomy is not usually necessary, but it has to be considered depending on the localization (esophagogastric junction) and/or extension of the tumor.

The rectal GISTs are uncommon and their definitive diagnosis is frequently obtained after the anatomopathological study of the surgical specimen. The rectal GIST of small dimensions, located in lower third, can be removed with complete parietal resection, through a transanal or transsphincteric procedure. However, these type of procedures must be performed with due care, because there are lower R0 resections (32% *versus* 82%) and higher rates of local recurrence (77% *versus* 31%), when compared with the previous lower anterior rectal resections, that is the procedure recommended for GISTs of the upper and middle thirds of the rectum (Changchien, Wu et al. 2004; Dong, Jun-Hui et al. 2007).

The surgical technique used to resect GISTs has implications in the occurrence of tumoral recurrence. The rupture of the tumor must be strictly prevented in all the GIST cases, especially in those which have great cystic or necrotic areas. The enucleation of the GISTs is considered an insufficient option, because it can easily not remove part of the pseudo-capsule, with persistence of viable tumor cells; on the other hand, it also associates with more frequent tumoral rupture. For these reasons, the enucleation is not recommended, even when the objective is to preserve a vital structure (Nishimura, Nakajima et al. 2007).

When the GIST develops and presents great dimensions, it can be submitted to a pre-surgical (neoadjuvant) treatment with imatinib, aiming to get better conditions of resectability of a tumor that is, many times, necrotic and friable (Eisenberg, Harris et al. 2009). This option can facilitate the complete surgical resection associated to tumor response to the treatment (Fig. 1), and/or the preservation of the function or the organ, particularly in GISTs of the esophagogastric junction, the second portion of the duodenum and the lower rectum (Casali and Blay 2010; Demetri, von Mehren et al. 2010). When there is invasion of adjacent organs, *en bloc* resection can be an alternative (Fig. 2). However, it is generally accepted that an incomplete resection of the tumor must be only performed as a palliative therapeutic option, in cases of hemorrhage, pain or symptoms secondary to the mass effect of the tumor.

When the R0 surgical resection is predicted to result in functional complications or important co-morbidities, and the neoadjuvant medical treatment was not efficient or cannot be given, the decision to carry a R1 resection must be discussed with the patient. The R1 resection can be acceptable in GISTs of low risk. There are no studies that clearly demonstrate the association between R1 surgery and shorter survival of the patients (Hohenberger and Eisenberg 2010).

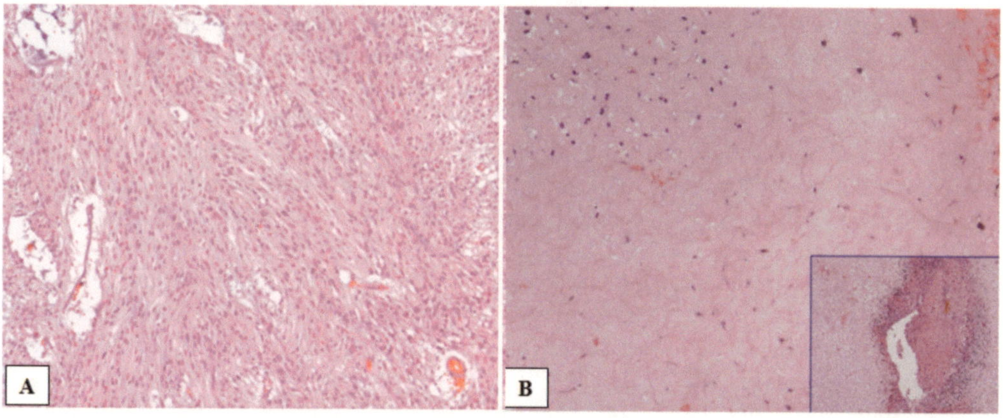

Fig. 1. GIST: biopsy microscopic features of an unresectable tumor (A); the tumor was submitted to a R0 resection after neoadjuvant imatinib (B). Note the substantial decreasing of the tumor cells density (B) with abundant sclero-hyaline stroma and hemorrhagic areas (inset) compared to pre-imatinib features (A).

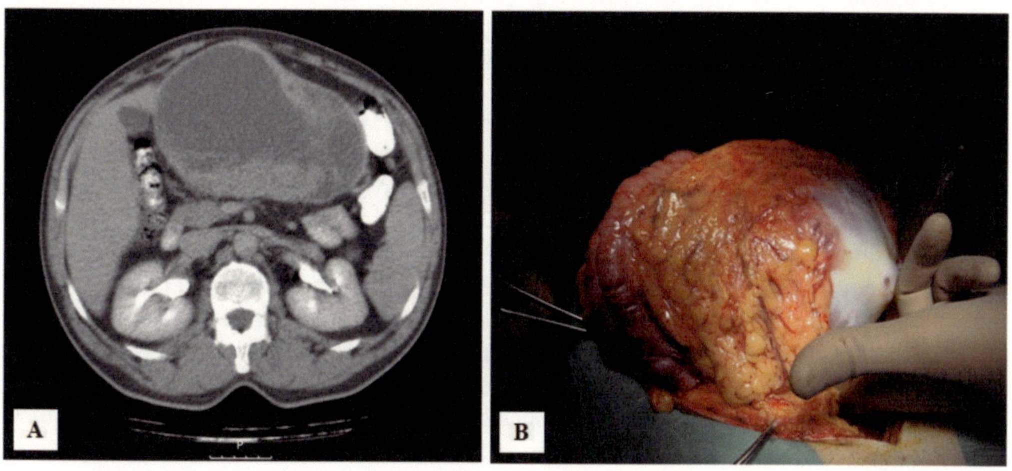

Fig. 2. GIST: CT scan of a large dimension GIST invading adjacent transverse colon (A); macroscopic aspect of the surgical specimen with R0 resection (B).

Many authors described that GISTs metastasize rarely for the lymph nodes, even in high risk cases. Bucher *et al.* (Bucher, Egger et al. 2006) described that 5 out of 80 patients (6%) with localized GIST developed hematogenous metastases, with or without lymph node involvement. In the series of Rutkowski *et al.* (Rutkowski, Nowecki et al. 2007), that include 335 patients, only four cases (1.2%) disclosed metastatic lymph nodes. The published studies indicate that there is no evidence of benefit for routine lymphadenectomy in the surgical treatment of GISTs, except when there is macroscopic lymph node involvement by the tumor (DeMatteo, Lewis et al. 2000; van der Zwan and DeMatteo 2005; Bucher, Egger et al. 2006; Otani, Furukawa et al. 2006; Casali and Blay 2010; Demetri, von Mehren et al. 2010).

3. Laparoscopic surgery

The laparoscopic surgery in GISTs is gradually expanding and being more used in recent years. The endoscopic diagnosis improved the capacity to identify gastric GISTs of small dimensions that are associated with a low risk of aggressiveness (Fletcher, Berman et al. 2002; Miettinen and Lasota 2006). The minimally invasive approach has become generally used in these tumors, due to the potential benefits of preventing the laparotomy of the patients. One should follow the strict oncologic principles of the open surgery: complete resection of the tumor with free margins (R0), preventing the dissemination of tumor cells into the peritoneal cavity (Otani and Kitajima 2005; Casali and Blay 2010; Demetri, von Mehren et al. 2010). In the GISTs of large dimensions, R1 resection can be complicated by rupture due to manipulation of the tumor and peritoneal dissemination. Therefore, laparoscopic resection has been discouraged in patients with GISTs of great dimensions (Blay, Bonvalot et al. 2005; Hohenberger and Eisenberg 2010). However, Novitsky *et al.* (Novitsky, Kercher et al. 2006) suggested that these recommendations should be reviewed, because they were not based on evidence but only translated precaution for the inexperienced surgeons with this procedure, aiming over all to prevent the increase of the incidence of tumor rupture. Several authors proposed the adoption of widened indications for the laparoscopic surgery in GISTs (Mochizuki, Kodera et al. 2004; Mochizuki, Kodera et al. 2006). Several studies described the accomplishment of laparoscopic resection of tumors with dimensions between 0.3 and 12.5 cm (Catena, Di Battista et al. 2008; Hohenberger and Eisenberg 2010), supplying evidence for the application of this procedure mainly in gastric GISTs. However, there are no controlled randomized studies in prospective clinical trials concluded to date to validate these options.

In the NCCN 2007 update, it is considered acceptable the laparoscopic resection of tumors > 5 cm, depending on the localization and the morphology, using laparoscopic or hand-assisted techniques (Novitsky, Kercher et al. 2006; Demetri, Benjamin et al. 2007; Catena, Di Battista et al. 2008; Demetri, von Mehren et al. 2010).

Before initiating the resection of the tumor, a formal throughout exploration of the abdominal cavity must be carried out to exclude the eventual presence of peritoneal or liver metastases. The use of ultrasound during surgery can be useful in the evaluation of possible liver metastases, and in case of suspected lesions, to guide the accomplishment of their biopsies. The use of intraoperative flexible endoscopy has been also frequently used to assist in more precise localization of small dimension GISTs and in the selection of the most adequate technique for the resection in the individual case. To prevent the risk of tumor rupture occurrence, GISTs should not be directly manipulated with the laparoscopic instruments (Novitsky, Kercher et al. 2006). Although there are no available evidence based data, the use of a bag for the removal of the surgical specimen seems to be essential to prevent the dissemination of tumor cells into the abdominal cavity or in the orifice of the laparoscopic port, and eventually metastases (Novitsky, Kercher et al. 2006; Ronellenfitsch, Staiger et al. 2009; Casali and Blay 2010).

For the treatment of gastric GISTs, different procedures have been used in the diverse published series, depending on several factors (e.g., dimension, localization and macroscopic features of the tumor): wedge or segmental resections using laparoscopy, laparoendoscopy (intragastric) or hand-assisted laparoscopy. The GISTs of the anterior wall and of the lesser and greater curvatures of the stomach are generally submitted to wedge resection, with linear endoscopic GI anastomosis stapler. The tumors of larger dimensions can be resected with free margins, using the ultrasonic coagulating shears (Novitsky, Kercher et al. 2006). The tumors of the posterior wall are many times removed via the lesser sac, but the transgastric approach, with anterior gastrotomy, constitutes a valid alternative, especially in the GISTs located next to the esophagogastric junction (Matthews, Walsh et al. 2002; Ludwig, Weiner et al. 2003; Li, Hung et al. 2008; Privette, McCahill et al. 2008). This option is, however, technically demanding and there are reports of incomplete resections and postoperative complications, such as stenosis and leakage in the suture line. The combined intragastric endoscopic-laparoscopic resection has been described as an alternative method in the treatment of the esophagogastric junction GISTs (Novitsky, Kercher et al. 2006; Ronellenfitsch, Staiger et al. 2009).

The localization of the tumor does not have to be considered an absolute contraindication for minimally invasive surgery, whenever the experience necessary for the technique and all the indispensable precautions are considered. However, in GISTs with large dimensions and/or with unfavorable localizations, as the gastric lesser curvature or the esophagogastric junction, it may not be possible to perform wedge resection with free tumor margins, being sometimes necessary to opt for subtotal or total gastrectomy. In these cases, the neoadjuvant treatment with imatinib, as suggested in the guidelines of ESMO and NCCN, may be a valid option to reduce the dimension of the tumor, and allow a resection with some preservation of the organ /function. However, the feasibility and the results of this type of procedures need validation from ongoing studies (Eisenberg 2006).

The laparoscopic surgery can be applied in other anatomic sites, such as rectal GISTs of small dimensions. However, the available data relative to the laparoscopic resections of GISTs in other (extra gastric) localizations are limited (Demetri, von Mehren et al. 2010).

The published global results of the laparoscopic surgery describe that the intraoperative and postoperative complications are relatively rare, occurring, respectively, in 6.8% and 7.7% of the patients (Hohenberger and Eisenberg 2010). The resections elapse with minimum losses of blood, satisfying the duration of surgery and short periods of hospital stay (Catena, Di Battista et al. 2008; Ronellenfitsch, Staiger et al. 2009). The morbidity related with the surgical wound of laparotomy is also prevented. The learning curve in the laparoscopic procedures indicates that, with better technical experience, the surgical times will be gradually improved (Shin 2005; Avital, Hermon et al. 2006).

Although the follow-up data of the patients are scarce, not exceeding ~ 5 years of duration (Hohenberger and Eisenberg 2010), some series described similar oncologic efficacy in the laparoscopic procedures when compared with those obtained with conventional surgery (Otani, Ohgami et al. 2000; Novitsky, Kercher et al. 2006; Choi, Kim et al. 2007)

The applicability of the laparoscopic approach must, therefore, be based in a variety of factors, including the characteristics of patient, dimension and the macroscopic morphology of the tumor, the pattern of invasion and the localization of the tumor, as well as the experience and qualification in laparoscopic surgery of the surgeon (Novitsky, Kercher et al. 2006).

The data from the literature indicate that laparoscopic resections or assisted by laparoscopy are feasible and associated with reduced rates of recurrence, short periods of internment and low morbidity (Otani, Ohgami et al. 2000; Novitsky, Kercher et al. 2006; Otani, Furukawa et al. 2006; Nishimura, Nakajima et al. 2007; Huguet, Rush et al. 2008; Nakamori, Iwahashi et al. 2008). This procedure must be recommended as the option of choice for the majority of patients with the small and intermediate dimension localized gastric GISTs.

4. Locally advanced primary GIST

In the advanced GISTs, without distant metastases, it can be impracticable the accomplishment of R0 resection. In these cases, it must be considered the tumoral cytoreduction with neoadjuvant imatinib. This option can facilitate the achievement of surgical R0 margins and allow a less extensive surgery, with better functional results, as suggested by the ESMO and the NCCN recommendations in such circumstances. However, these recommendations are based only on publications of retrospective non-randomized data (Shah, Sun et al. 2005; Goh, Chow et al. 2006). The primary treatment with imatinib for tumor cytoreduction can still be considered in GISTs whenever there is a high risk of hemorrhage or tumoral rupture during surgery.

The maximum therapeutic response is usually reached after 6-12 months of treatment. The subsequent surgical intervention can then be safely performed in the majority of the cases (Bumming, Andersson et al. 2003; Eisenberg, Harris et al. 2009; Casali and Blay 2010). However, it is not always necessary to wait for the maximum response to perform the surgery. The mutacional analysis of the tumor can assist to exclude from this therapeutic neoadjuvant option GISTs with lower response rates to imatinib (e.g., with *PDGFRA* D842V mutation), and/or allow to change for a more adequate therapeutic option. A PET or PET/CT, or the evaluation of the tumor density with CT scan, can be particularly useful in the early evaluation of tumor response to the therapeutic option, without delaying the surgical intervention in GISTs that do not respond to the treatment (Townsend, Carney et al. 2004; Goldstein, Tan et al. 2005; Heinicke, Wardelmann et al. 2005; Dimitrakopoulou-Strauss, Hohenberger et al. 2007).

It is essential to establish a multidisciplinary therapeutic decision plan (tumor conference) involving several specialties, including pathologists, oncologists, radiologists, gastroenterologists, and surgeons. The sharing of experiences, available in reference centers for sarcomas, including GISTs, and/or in oncologic networks to assist patients, must be considered as an essential condition for the adequate individual management of patients with GISTs (Casali and Blay 2010).

5. Conclusion

Gastrointestinal stromal tumors (GISTs) are the most common gastrointestinal tract (GI) mesenchymal tumors. GIST diagnosis must be confirmed by immunohistochemistry, rarely by molecular study, and integrated with other clinical and morphological features. Biological behavior is uncertain and classification (including largest size, mitotic rate and GI site) in risk categories is useful for predicting clinical behavior of GISTs.

The definitive treatment of primary GISTs $\geq$ 2 cm without peritoneal dissemination or distant metastases is complete macroscopic surgical resection. Some authors sustain that the microscopic status (R1 or R0) of the surgical margins does not influences survival, or even recurrence of GISTs, while others suggest that R0 resections may influence the prognosis of patients. In our experience, the recurrence rate is significantly lower in R0 cases, but in the multivariate analysis only R2 is significantly associated with shorter disease specific survival of patients with GIST. R1 resection may expose patients to a higher risk of tumor locoregional recurrence. The gold standard of ESMO and NCCN recommendations for surgery of GIST is complete (R0) resection without tumor rupture.

Surgical procedures can change, depending on the involved organ, its precise site, and the dimension of GIST. Wedge resection is the most frequent option for GISTs in the stomach, and segmental resection for those in the small bowel. For large dimension tumors in the gastric lesser curvature and/or with pyloric involvement, a distal gastrectomy may be better option, and total gastrectomy may be also considered, depending on the site (esophagogastric junction) and/or extension of the GIST. There is no evidence of benefit for routine lymphadenectomy in the surgical treatment of GISTs.

The minimally invasive approach is being commonly used in gastric tumors, avoiding laparotomy of patients. Nevertheless, controlled randomized studies in prospective clinical trials are warranted to validate this option. Worth mentioning, one should follow in this approach the same stringent oncologic standards of open surgery: complete resection (R0) of the tumor, avoiding dissemination into the peritoneal cavity. The NCCN 2007 update considers suitable the laparoscopic resection of tumors > 5 cm, depending on the site and the morphology, using laparoscopic or hand-assisted techniques. Laparoscopic resections or assisted by laparoscopy are feasible with reduced rates of recurrence, short periods of internment, and low morbidity.

In locally advanced GISTs, without distant metastases, tumor cytoreduction with neoadjuvant imatinib can enable R0 margins and less mutilating surgery, with better functional results, as proposed by the retrospective non-randomized based data included in ESMO and NCCN recommendations. The mutational analysis of the tumor can assist to exclude from the neoadjuvant option GISTs with lower response rates to imatinib (e.g., with *PDGFRA* D842V mutation), and/or allow a more adequate available therapeutic option.

Considering the persisting controversies, it is essential to set up a multidisciplinary therapeutic decision plan involving several specialties. The input of experiences, available in reference centers for sarcomas, in addition to the patient involvement and informed consent, must be considered as standard of care conditions for the adequate individual management of GISTs.

6. References

Agaimy, A., L. M. Terracciano, et al. (2009). "V600E BRAF mutations are alternative early molecular events in a subset of KIT/PDGFRA wild-type gastrointestinal stromal tumours." J Clin Pathol 62(7): 613-6.

Agaram, N. P., G. C. Wong, et al. (2008). "Novel V600E BRAF mutations in imatinib-naive and imatinib-resistant gastrointestinal stromal tumors." Genes Chromosomes Cancer 47(10): 853-9.

Ahmed, I., N. T. Welch, et al. (2008). "Gastrointestinal stromal tumours (GIST) - 17 years experience from Mid Trent Region (United Kingdom)." Eur J Surg Oncol 34(4): 445-9.

Aparicio, T., V. Boige, et al. (2004). "Prognostic factors after surgery of primary resectable gastrointestinal stromal tumours." Eur J Surg Oncol 30(10): 1098-103.

Avital, S., H. Hermon, et al. (2006). "Learning curve in laparoscopic colorectal surgery: our first 100 patients." Isr Med Assoc J 8(10): 683-6.

Blay, J. Y., S. Bonvalot, et al. (2005). "Consensus meeting for the management of gastrointestinal stromal tumors. Report of the GIST Consensus Conference of 20-21 March 2004, under the auspices of ESMO." Ann Oncol 16(4): 566-78.

Boni, L., A. Benevento, et al. (2005). "Surgical resection for gastrointestinal stromal tumors (GIST): experience on 25 patients." World J Surg Oncol 3: 78.

Bucher, P., J. F. Egger, et al. (2006). "An audit of surgical management of gastrointestinal stromal tumours (GIST)." Eur J Surg Oncol 32(3): 310-4.

Bucher, P., S. Taylor, et al. (2004). "Are there any prognostic factors for small intestinal stromal tumors?" Am J Surg 187(6): 761-6.

Bumming, P., H. Ahlman, et al. (2006). "Population-based study of the diagnosis and treatment of gastrointestinal stromal tumours." Br J Surg 93(7): 836-43.

Bumming, P., J. Andersson, et al. (2003). "Neoadjuvant, adjuvant and palliative treatment of gastrointestinal stromal tumours (GIST) with imatinib: a centre-based study of 17 patients." Br J Cancer 89(3): 460-4.

Casali, P. G. and J. Y. Blay (2010). "Gastrointestinal stromal tumours: ESMO Clinical Practice Guidelines for diagnosis, treatment and follow-up." Ann Oncol 21 Suppl 5: v98-102.

Catena, F., M. Di Battista, et al. (2008). "Laparoscopic treatment of gastric GIST: report of 21 cases and literature's review." J Gastrointest Surg 12(3): 561-8.

Changchien, C. R., M. C. Wu, et al. (2004). "Evaluation of prognosis for malignant rectal gastrointestinal stromal tumor by clinical parameters and immunohistochemical staining." Dis Colon Rectum 47(11): 1922-9.

Choi, S. M., M. C. Kim, et al. (2007). "Laparoscopic wedge resection for gastric GIST: long-term follow-up results." Eur J Surg Oncol 33(4): 444-7.

Connolly, E. M., E. Gaffney, et al. (2003). "Gastrointestinal stromal tumours." Br J Surg 90(10): 1178-86.

Corless, C. L. and M. C. Heinrich (2008). "Molecular pathobiology of gastrointestinal stromal sarcomas." Annu Rev Pathol 3: 557-86.

Crosby, J. A., C. N. Catton, et al. (2001). "Malignant gastrointestinal stromal tumors of the small intestine: a review of 50 cases from a prospective database." Ann Surg Oncol 8(1): 50-9.

Dematteo, R. P., M. C. Heinrich, et al. (2002). "Clinical management of gastrointestinal stromal tumors: before and after STI-571." Hum Pathol 33(5): 466-77.

DeMatteo, R. P., J. J. Lewis, et al. (2000). "Two hundred gastrointestinal stromal tumors: recurrence patterns and prognostic factors for survival." Ann Surg 231(1): 51-8.

Demetri, G. D., L. H. Baker, et al. (2007). "Soft tissue sarcoma." J Natl Compr Canc Netw 5(4): 364-99.

Demetri, G. D., R. S. Benjamin, et al. (2007). "NCCN Task Force report: management of patients with gastrointestinal stromal tumor (GIST)--update of the NCCN clinical practice guidelines." J Natl Compr Canc Netw 5 Suppl 2: S1-29; quiz S30.

Demetri, G. D., M. von Mehren, et al. (2010). "NCCN Task Force report: update on the management of patients with gastrointestinal stromal tumors." J Natl Compr Canc Netw 8 Suppl 2: S1-41; quiz S42-4.

Dimitrakopoulou-Strauss, A., P. Hohenberger, et al. (2007). "68Ga-labeled bombesin studies in patients with gastrointestinal stromal tumors: comparison with 18F-FDG." J Nucl Med 48(8): 1245-50.

Dong, C., C. Jun-Hui, et al. (2007). "Gastrointestinal stromal tumors of the rectum: Clinical, pathologic, immunohistochemical characteristics and prognostic analysis." Scand J Gastroenterol 42(10): 1221-9.

Eisenberg, B. L. (2006). "Combining imatinib with surgery in gastrointestinal stromal tumors: rationale and ongoing trials." Clin Colorectal Cancer 6 Suppl 1: S24-9.

Eisenberg, B. L., J. Harris, et al. (2009). "Phase II trial of neoadjuvant/adjuvant imatinib mesylate (IM) for advanced primary and metastatic/recurrent operable gastrointestinal stromal tumor (GIST): early results of RTOG 0132/ACRIN 6665." J Surg Oncol 99(1): 42-7.

Eisenberg, B. L. and I. Judson (2004). "Surgery and imatinib in the management of GIST: emerging approaches to adjuvant and neoadjuvant therapy." Ann Surg Oncol 11(5): 465-75.

Fletcher, C. D., J. J. Berman, et al. (2002). "Diagnosis of gastrointestinal stromal tumors: A consensus approach." Hum Pathol 33(5): 459-65.

Fujimoto, Y., Y. Nakanishi, et al. (2003). "Clinicopathologic study of primary malignant gastrointestinal stromal tumor of the stomach, with special reference to prognostic factors: analysis of results in 140 surgically resected patients." Gastric Cancer 6(1): 39-48.

Gajiwala, K. S., J. C. Wu, et al. (2009). "KIT kinase mutants show unique mechanisms of drug resistance to imatinib and sunitinib in gastrointestinal stromal tumor patients." Proc Natl Acad Sci U S A 106(5): 1542-7.

Goh, B. K., P. K. Chow, et al. (2006). "Pathologic, radiologic and PET scan response of gastrointestinal stromal tumors after neoadjuvant treatment with imatinib mesylate." Eur J Surg Oncol 32(9): 961-3.

Goldstein, D., B. S. Tan, et al. (2005). "Gastrointestinal stromal tumours: correlation of F-FDG gamma camera-based coincidence positron emission tomography with CT for the assessment of treatment response--an AGITG study." Oncology 69(4): 326-32.

Gomes, A. L., A. Gouveia, et al. (2008). "Molecular alterations of KIT and PDGFRA in GISTs: evaluation of a Portuguese series." J Clin Pathol 61(2): 203-8.

Gouveia, A. M., A. P. Pimenta, et al. (2008). "Surgical margin status and prognosis of gastrointestinal stromal tumor." World J Surg 32(11): 2375-82.

He, L. J., B. S. Wang, et al. (1988). "Smooth muscle tumours of the digestive tract: report of 160 cases." Br J Surg 75(2): 184-6.

Heinicke, T., E. Wardelmann, et al. (2005). "Very early detection of response to imatinib mesylate therapy of gastrointestinal stromal tumours using 18fluoro-deoxyglucose-positron emission tomography." Anticancer Res 25(6C): 4591-4.

Heinrich, M. C. and C. L. Corless (2005). "Gastric GI stromal tumors (GISTs): the role of surgery in the era of targeted therapy." J Surg Oncol 90(3): 195-207; discussion 207.

Heinrich, M. C., C. L. Corless, et al. (2003). "Kinase mutations and imatinib response in patients with metastatic gastrointestinal stromal tumor." J Clin Oncol 21(23): 4342-9.

Hinz, S., U. Pauser, et al. (2006). "Audit of a series of 40 gastrointestinal stromal tumour cases." Eur J Surg Oncol 32(10): 1125-9.

Hoeben, A., P. Schoffski, et al. (2008). "Clinical implications of mutational analysis in gastrointestinal stromal tumours." Br J Cancer 98(4): 684-8.

Hohenberger, P. and B. Eisenberg (2010). "Role of Surgery Combined with Kinase Inhibition in the Management of Gastrointestinal Stromal Tumor (GIST)." Ann Surg Oncol.

Hostein, I., N. Faur, et al. (2010). "BRAF mutation status in gastrointestinal stromal tumors." Am J Clin Pathol 133(1): 141-8.

Howe, J. R., L. H. Karnell, et al. (2001). "Small bowel sarcoma: analysis of survival from the National Cancer Data Base." Ann Surg Oncol 8(6): 496-508.

Huguet, K. L., R. M. Rush, Jr., et al. (2008). "Laparoscopic gastric gastrointestinal stromal tumor resection: the mayo clinic experience." Arch Surg 143(6): 587-90; discussion 591.

Langer, C., B. Gunawan, et al. (2003). "Prognostic factors influencing surgical management and outcome of gastrointestinal stromal tumours." Br J Surg 90(3): 332-9.

Lehnert, T. (1998). "Gastrointestinal sarcoma (GIST)--a review of surgical management." Ann Chir Gynaecol 87(4): 297-305.

Li, V. K., W. K. Hung, et al. (2008). "Laparoscopic intragastric approach for stromal tumours located at the posterior gastric wall." Asian J Surg 31(1): 6-10.

Liegl-Atzwanger, B., J. A. Fletcher, et al. (2010). "Gastrointestinal stromal tumors." Virchows Arch 456(2): 111-27.

Lin, S. C., M. J. Huang, et al. (2003). "Clinical manifestations and prognostic factors in patients with gastrointestinal stromal tumors." World J Gastroenterol 9(12): 2809-12.

Lok, K. H., L. Lai, et al. (2009). "Endosonographic surveillance of small gastrointestinal tumors originating from muscularis propria." J Gastrointestin Liver Dis 18(2): 177-80.

Ludwig, K., R. Weiner, et al. (2003). "[Minimally invasive resections of gastric tumors]." Chirurg 74(7): 632-7.

Martinho, O., A. Gouveia, et al. (2009). "Loss of RKIP expression is associated with poor survival in GISTs." Virchows Arch 455(3): 277-84.

Martinho, O., A. Gouveia, et al. (2009). "Low frequency of MAP kinase pathway alterations in KIT and PDGFRA wild-type GISTs." Histopathology 55(1): 53-62.

Matthews, B. D., R. M. Walsh, et al. (2002). "Laparoscopic vs open resection of gastric stromal tumors." Surg Endosc 16(5): 803-7.

Mazur, M. T. and H. B. Clark (1983). "Gastric stromal tumors. Reappraisal of histogenesis." Am J Surg Pathol 7(6): 507-19.

Miettinen, M. and J. Lasota (2006). "Gastrointestinal stromal tumors: pathology and prognosis at different sites." Semin Diagn Pathol 23(2): 70-83.

Mochizuki, Y., Y. Kodera, et al. (2006). "Laparoscopic wedge resection for gastrointestinal stromal tumors of the stomach: initial experience." Surg Today 36(4): 341-7.

Mochizuki, Y., Y. Kodera, et al. (2004). "Treatment and risk factors for recurrence after curative resection of gastrointestinal stromal tumors of the stomach." World J Surg 28(9): 870-5.

Nakamori, M., M. Iwahashi, et al. (2008). "Laparoscopic resection for gastrointestinal stromal tumors of the stomach." Am J Surg 196(3): 425-9.

Ng, E. H., R. E. Pollock, et al. (1992). "Prognostic factors influencing survival in gastrointestinal leiomyosarcomas. Implications for surgical management and staging." Ann Surg 215(1): 68-77.

Nishimura, J., K. Nakajima, et al. (2007). "Surgical strategy for gastric gastrointestinal stromal tumors: laparoscopic vs. open resection." Surg Endosc 21(6): 875-8.

Novitsky, Y. W., K. W. Kercher, et al. (2006). "Long-term outcomes of laparoscopic resection of gastric gastrointestinal stromal tumors." Ann Surg 243(6): 738-45; discussion 745-7.

Otani, Y., T. Furukawa, et al. (2006). "Operative indications for relatively small (2-5 cm) gastrointestinal stromal tumor of the stomach based on analysis of 60 operated cases." Surgery 139(4): 484-92.

Otani, Y. and M. Kitajima (2005). "Laparoscopic surgery for GIST: too soon to decide." Gastric Cancer 8(3): 135-6.

Otani, Y., M. Ohgami, et al. (2000). "Laparoscopic wedge resection of gastric submucosal tumors." Surg Laparosc Endosc Percutan Tech 10(1): 19-23.

Pidhorecky, I., R. T. Cheney, et al. (2000). "Gastrointestinal stromal tumors: current diagnosis, biologic behavior, and management." Ann Surg Oncol 7(9): 705-12.

Pierie, J. P., U. Choudry, et al. (2001). "The effect of surgery and grade on outcome of gastrointestinal stromal tumors." Arch Surg 136(4): 383-9.

Privette, A., L. McCahill, et al. (2008). "Laparoscopic approaches to resection of suspected gastric gastrointestinal stromal tumors based on tumor location." Surg Endosc 22(2): 487-94.

Ronellenfitsch, U., W. Staiger, et al. (2009). "Perioperative and oncological outcome of laparoscopic resection of gastrointestinal stromal tumour (GIST) of the stomach." Diagn Ther Endosc 2009: 286138.

Rutkowski, P., Z. I. Nowecki, et al. (2007). "Risk criteria and prognostic factors for predicting recurrences after resection of primary gastrointestinal stromal tumor." Ann Surg Oncol 14(7): 2018-27.

Shah, J. N., W. Sun, et al. (2005). "Neoadjuvant therapy with imatinib mesylate for locally advanced GI stromal tumor." Gastrointest Endosc 61(4): 625-7.

Shin, R. B. (2005). "Evaluation of the learning curve for laparoscopic Roux-en-Y gastric bypass surgery." Surg Obes Relat Dis 1(2): 91-4.

Townsend, D. W., J. P. Carney, et al. (2004). "PET/CT today and tomorrow." J Nucl Med 45 Suppl 1: 4S-14S.

van der Zwan, S. M. and R. P. DeMatteo (2005). "Gastrointestinal stromal tumor: 5 years later." Cancer 104(9): 1781-8.

Wardelmann, E., R. Buttner, et al. (2007). "Mutation analysis of gastrointestinal stromal tumors: increasing significance for risk assessment and effective targeted therapy." Virchows Arch 451(4): 743-9.

Wong, N. A., R. Young, et al. (2003). "Prognostic indicators for gastrointestinal stromal tumours: a clinicopathological and immunohistochemical study of 108 resected cases of the stomach." Histopathology 43(2): 118-26.

Wu, P. C., A. Langerman, et al. (2003). "Surgical treatment of gastrointestinal stromal tumors in the imatinib (STI-571) era." Surgery 134(4): 656-65; discussion 665-6.

Wu, T. J., L. Y. Lee, et al. (2006). "Surgical treatment and prognostic analysis for gastrointestinal stromal tumors (GISTs) of the small intestine: before the era of imatinib mesylate." BMC Gastroenterol 6: 29.

Yan, H., P. Marchettini, et al. (2003). "Prognostic assessment of gastrointestinal stromal tumor." Am J Clin Oncol 26(3): 221-8.

5

The Role of the Surgeon in Multidisciplinary Approach to Gastrointestinal Stromal Tumors

Selim Sözen[1], Ömer Topuz[2] and
Yasemin Benderli Cihan[3]
[1]*Adana Numune Training And Research Hospital General Surgery Department, Adana*
[2]*Kayseri Training And Research Hospital General Surgery Department, Kayseri*
[3]*Kayseri Training And Research Hospital Radiation Oncology Department, Kayseri*
Turkey

1. Introduction

Gastrointestinal stromal tumours (GISTs) are the most common mesenchymal neoplasms of the digestive tract with an estimated annual incidence of 10–20 cases per one million inhabitants (H. Joensuu et al;2002, B. Nilsson, et al; 2005). GISTs probably arise from precursor cells of the interstitial cells of Cajal. Their defining characteristic is a gain-of-function mutation in genes coding for the KIT tyrosine kinase receptor, which is considered the driving force of cell proliferation in this tumour(Y. Shinomura et al;2005) Gastrointestinal stromal tumors usually appear in patients above 50 years of age, whereas the maximum incidence is observed in the 5th and the 6th decade of life. The mean age at the diagnosis is 55–63 years(Tran T et al; 2005). It is very rare in children and affects males and females equally. GIST is mainly a disease of the GI tract, mesentery, and omentum. Most commonly, it originates in the stomach (60%), followed by the small intestine (30%), the colon and rectum (5%), and the oesophagus (5%) (Van Der Zwan SM, et al;2005). Fletcher et al. proposed a classification of aggressive behaviour for GISTs based on their maximum diameter and mitotic rate(C. D. M. Fletcher et al;2002). factors which were both shown to predict recurrence and survival(S. Singer et al;2002, R. P. DeMatteo et al;2000). GIST can present in many ways. Thirty percent are diagnosed incidentally on a pathological or autopsy resection specimen(B. Nilsson, et al; 2005). Small tumors may be asymptomatic and GISTs can grow to a large size before producing any symptoms. Most symptomatic patients present with tumours larger than 5 cm in maximal dimension. Symptoms at presentation may include abdominal pain, abdominal mass, nausea, vomiting, anorexia, and weight loss. The vast majority of metastatic GISTs are located intraabdominal, either in the liver, in the omentum, or in the peritoneal cavity(C. D. M. Fletcher et al;2002). Metastatic spread to lymph nodes and to other regions via lymphatics is very rare. Most of the patients with GIST are symptomatic and bleding due to mucosal ulceration is the most common symptom(Gold JS et al ; 2006). Mitotic count and tumor size have been shown to be very important. A large study examined 1765 tumors for prognostic markers(Miettinen et al; 2005). Tumours less than 10 cm with less than 5 mitoses per 50 high powered fields (HPFs) had only a 2%-3% risk of metastases. Conversely, the metastatic rate for tumors greater than 10 cm, with greater than 5 mitoses per 50 HPFs, was as high as 86%. Non-gastric primary tumor location and male gender may also be independent adverseprognostic factors(Rutkowski et al; 2007). Fletcher et al. proposed a classification of aggressive behaviour for GISTs based on their maximum diameter and mitotic rate(C. D. M. Fletcher et al;2002), factors which were both shown to predict recurrence and survival(S. Singer et al;2002, R. P. DeMatteo et al;2000). Surgery remains the standard initial management for all localized GIST. The tumor should be removed en bloc, with a clear margin. The pseudocapsule should be removed and not penetrated. Therefore, a wedge resection (stomach) or segmental resection (intestine) is required. If neighboring structures are involved, en-bloc resection should still be contemplated. It is mandatory that the resection achieves negative margins verified by intraoperative frozen section examination, since the presence of residual disease negatively influences survival(S. Singer et al;2002). The 5-year survival rate after surgery amounts to 28-65%(Debol SM et al;2001 ,Blay JY et al;2005). It is not necessary to resect the regional lymph nodes during the operation, because gastrointestinal stromal tumors do not metastasize to the regional lymphatic system.

2. Surgery

Primary GIST may occur anywhere along the GI tract from the esophagus to the anus(Judson I et al; 2002). The most frequent site is the stomach (55%), followed by the duodenum and small intestine (30%), esophagus (5%), rectum (5%), colon(2%), and rare other locations.

2.1 Treatment of the non-metastatic disease approach to the primary lesion (stomach)

The radical surgical treatment is the most effective treatment option for GIST. The 5-year survival rate after surgery amounts to 28-65%(R. P. DeMatteo et al;2000). It is not necessary to resect the regional lymph nodes during the operation, because gastrointestinal stromal tumors do not metastasize to the regional lymphatic system. Lymphatic metastasis rarely occurs (0-3.4%) in patients with GIST(Tashiro T et al; 2005). It is mandatory that the resection achieves negative margins verified by intraoperative frozen section examination, since the presence of residual disease negatively influences survival(S. Singer et al;2002). More recently, there has been a move to laparoscopic surgery, particularly for gastric GIST. One series of 50 consecutive patients showed this approach was associated with low morbidity and short hospitalization. All resections had clear margins and the long term disease free survival was 92%(Novitsky YW et al;2006). Current recommendation is that laparoscopy should be restricted to the treatment of small lesions (up to 5 cm) due to the possibility of tumor rupture as a result of the manipulation of larger lesions(Guitierrez JC et al;2007). Current NCCN guidelines do not contain a clear statement on whether surgery for GIST should be performed laparoscopically or through open surgery but recommend that surgery should produce minimal surgical morbidity(National Comprehensive Cancer Network (NCCN);2008). Recently, a new technique of endoscopic full-thickness resection using a flexible stapler was described. This approach seems particularly useful in tumours of the posterior distal part of the stomach(G. Kaehler et al;2006).

2.2 Treatment of the non-metastatic disease approach to the primary lesion (small intestine, duodenum and esophageal GISTs)

GISTs of the small intestine with histopathologic features including mitotic counts >5/50 HPF, high cellularity, absence of a predominant organoid growth pattern, absence of skeinoid fibers, presence of severe nuclear pleomorphism, presence of mucosal infilatration, and tumor cell necrosis have been significantly associated with an adverse outcome in the literature (Tworedk JA et al; 1997, Chang MS et al;1998). The treatment of choice is the complete resection of the tumour.(Figure 2) With regard to local invasion and tumor perforation, a tumor that has invaded a contiguous organ is considered to be advanced and associated with poor outcome(Shiu MH et al;1982, Ng EH et al;1992). Local invasion and tumor perforation were associated with poor DFS; although all gross disease was removed, these conditions were similar to those that occur with incomplete resections. Unlike therapy of mucosa and submocasa derived duodenum tumor, pancreas or duodenum resection is not required in therapy of duodenal stromal tumor which is tumorectomy. Unique treatment option of duodenal GIST is not Pancreatico-duodenectomy. Pancreas preserving segmental duodenum resection may be useful, comfortable and safe especially for the third

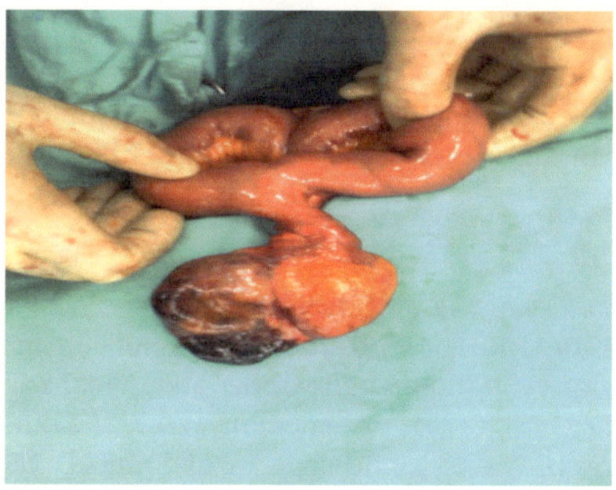

Fig. 1. Intraoperative picture showing tumour and Meckel's diverticulum. (Archived by SELİM SÖZEN)

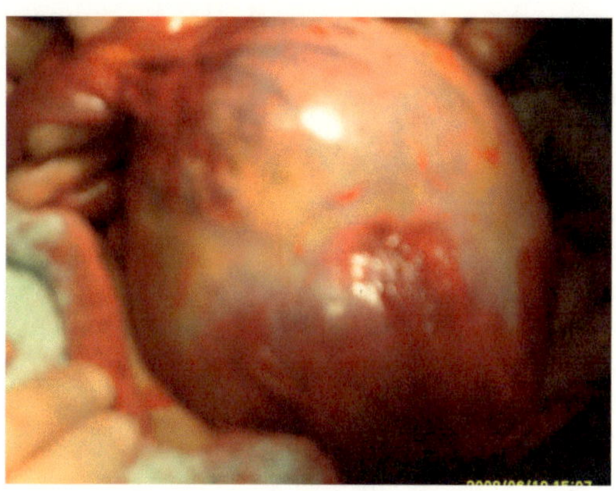

Fig. 2. The well-circumscribed lesion of the ileum before its removal. (Archived by SELİM SÖZEN)

part GIST of duodenum. Esophageal tumors are usually small and asymptomatic, larger lesions present with dysphagia, and sometimes they may be found accidentally, as an abnormal mediastinal shadow on chest X-ray. Relevant literature reports only a few cases of these kinds of tumors, some treated with esophageal resection and others treated with enucleation (Spinelli GP et al;2008).

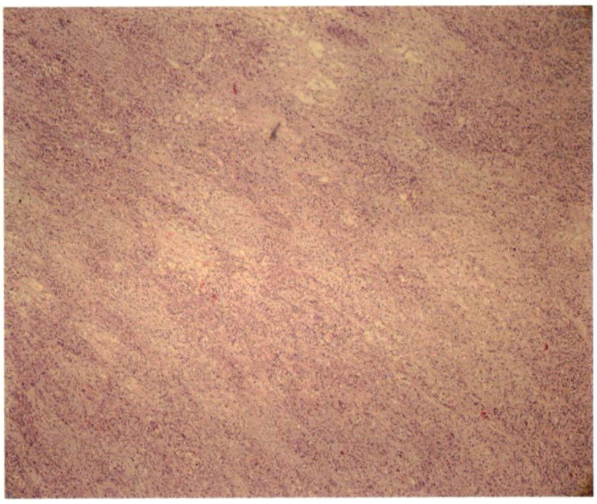

Fig. 3. Histopathology slide after Immunostaining for C-Kit; Tumour cells show positivity after C-Kit staining, which suggests GIST. (Archived by SELİM SÖZEN)

3. Small intestine

The clinical presentation is variable and depends on tumor size and anatomic site. Their submucosal location can produce local obstructive symptoms, particularly when arising in the oesophagus or the small intestine. Vague upper abdominal pain, fullness, GI bleeding, palpable mass are other modes of presentation whereas sometimes they are found incidentally during barium studies, endoscopy or abdominal scans performed for other reasons(Roberto Logrono et al;2004). According to some authors, visceral obstruction is a rare occurrence even in the presence of extensive peritoneal metastatic disease(Burkill GJC et al;2003). Although the diagnostic procedure includes several examinations, such as barium examination of the gastrointestinal track, computer tomography and angiography(Fang SH et al;2004) , none of them can establish the correct diagnosis with 100% certainty. The preoperative percutaneous fine needle aspiration of the tumor for diagnostic purpose is not indicated because of the danger for potential intraperitoneal migration or tumor rupture (Fang SH et al;2004). Recently, several studies pointed out the significance of endoscopic ultrasound-guided fine-needle aspiration for the diagnosis of GIST with a reported accuracy of 89% (Eloubeidi MA, et al;2004). On the other hand, positron-emission tomography (PET) with 18F-fluoro-2-deoxy-D-glucose is a very useful tool for the postoperative follow-up of patients receiving imatinib(Gelibter A et al;2004). The treatment of choice for GISTs is the surgical excision of the tumor. All tumors must be completely resected (R0 resection), where possible, including the tissues that are infiltrated, while systemic lymph node dissection is not recommended by many authors(Chen TW et al; 2005, Aparicio T et al;2004). Complete surgical resection is connected with 48-65% five-year survival. Partial resection must only be performed in case of large tumors, for palliative purposes or for the control of symptoms or complications such as compression of other organs, hemorrhage, or pain(Connolly EM et al;2003). The clinical presentations of GISTs of small bowel are variable and depend on the tumor size and anatomic site. In the review of Miettinen and Lasota(Miettinen M et al;2006) the most common presentation of GIST is reported as GI bleeding. The tumors smaller than 2 cm in size are generally asymptomatic and larger tumors may present with upper abdominal pain, palpable intra abdominal mass, vomiting, weight loss, and perforation or rupture. Computed tomography or magnetic resonance investigation is useful in tumors larger than 2 centimeters(Lupescu IG et al;2007, Spivach A et al;1999, Abbas M et al;2008). Endoscopic examinations fail in the diagnosis of GISTs originated from the small intestine. The long term survival is 50% at best. These tumors are believed to be potentially malignant lesions with an average rate of 20-25% of gastric and 40-50% of small intestinal localization. Metastases commonly develop in the abdominal cavity and liver; rarely, in bones, soft tissues, and skin (Abbas M et al;2008,Bucher P et al;2006, Miettinen M et al;2006). Prognostic factors for GISTs are the age, anatomic location, mitotic rate, and tumor size(Bucher P et al;2006, Efremidou EI et al;2006). Chemotherapy and radiotherapy do not increase the survival time. Radiotherapy is indicated in intraperitoneal hemorrhage and maintaining analgesia in unresectable tumors. Imatinib, a selective inhibitor of tyrosinekinases, is a hope promising drug, which is the first effective treatment for non-resectable or metastatic GISTs. Furthermore, imatinib is indicated in intraperitoneal perforated or ruptured GIST due to the possibility of peritoneal soiling (Efremidou EI et al;2006, Karagülle E et al;2008).

4. Duodenum

Duodenal GIST usually present with vague abdominal pain(50%-70%) or they bleed into the lumen(20%-50%)(Sturgeon C et al;2003, DeMatteo RP et al;2000). Second part of the duodenum seems to be the common site of duodenal GIST and most of them will require pancreatoduodenectomy for complete resection(Winfield et al;2006). Completely resected GIST has a five year survival of 30%-80%(Casper ES; 2000). Incompletely resected tumors have a high recurrence rate(upto 90%). Historically Unresectable/metastatic GIST has a median survival of 12 months(Roberts PJ et al;2002). Imatinib mesylate, a specific tyrosikine kinase inhibitor has produced a paradigm shift in the treatment of GIST, due to the targeted molecular therapy. Imatinib produce sustained clinical response in more than 50% of the patients with advanced GIST and one year survival in these patients was 88%(Demetri GD et al;2002). Surgery with negative surgical margins and no tumor rupture is a necessary and adequate means of treating such tumors. Extensive lymph node dissection is unnecessary, because GISTs rarely metastasize to the regional lymph nodes(Pidhorechly I et al;2000, Emory TS et al;1999, Dematteo RP et al;2000, Pieri JPEN et al;2001). When technically feasible, this makes duodenal resection preferable to pancreatoduodenectomy(Uehara K et al,2001). However, the optimal surgical treatment for duodenal GISTs has never been fully assessed. Recent anatomical knowledge of the head of the pancreas(Sakamoto Y et al;2000) has facilitated various methods of pancreatic resection for low-grade malignancies (52,53,54 Nakagohri T et al;2000, Thayer SP et al;2002, Sakamoto Y et al; 2002), and duodenal resection preserving the pancreatic head can now be performed safely.

5. Colon and rectum

GISTs are an extremely rare subset of colonic tumors that are difficult to distinguish grossly from the commonly encountered adenocarcinoma. GISTs are found commonly in the stomach (60 - 70%) and small intestine (20 - 30%), and rarely in the colon and rectum (5 - 10%) and esophagus (less than 5%).(Graadt van Roggen JF et al;2001). When in a colonic location, about two thirds of these GISTs occur in the left or transverse colon(57 Miettien M et al;2000) . These tumours predominantly occur in middle aged or older persons, the median age at presentation being sixty years, and are uncommon below forty years of age(Graadt van Roggen JF et al;2001, Mukhopadyay S et al;2002). Males and females are affected equally, but a peculiar subset occurs in female patients below the age of 21 years, either singly or in association with pulmonary chondromas and extra-adrenal paraganglionomas (Carney's syndrome)(Graadt van Roggen JF et al;2001).

Grossly, GISTs may vary greatly in size. Smaller tumours (2 cm or less) are usually asymptomatic and are usually detected incidentally during investigations or at surgery for unrelated pathology. These often exhibit a benign nature, but at times, may present with metastasis to the liver and lungs(DeMatteo RP et al; 2000). Larger tumours usually behave like malignant tumors, and may present with abdominal pain and gastrointestinal bleeding due to ulceration of the overlying mucosa, abdominal mass, or with nonspecific symptoms such as weight loss, vomiting, fever and anemia. Depending on the site, the tumor may also present with obstruction, dysphagia, altered bowel habits, or rarely, obstructive jaundice(Burkill GJC et al;2003, Ludwig DJ et al;1997). Complete gross excision of the tumor is the treatment of choice; routine lymph node excision is not recommended since they are rarely involved. However, it must be stressed here that in the absence of a clear cut diagnosis of colonic GIST, surgery must proceed as if for adenocarcinoma and radical clearance should be done. Care must be taken to avoid tumour rupture during surgery, since this has been implicated as one of the causes of recurrence(Mukhopadyay S et al;2002, DeMatteo RP et al; 2000). Colorectal GISTs are relatively rare, frequency being reported at approximately 5%(Miettinen M et al;2000).Moreover, the pathobiological features of malignant GISTs of the colon remain unclear. Most rectal tumours are of epithelial origin. Only a small number of rectal tumours originate from the smooth muscle cells in the rectal wall. Such stromal tumours are either benign (leiomyoma) or show malignant characteristics (formerly known as leiomyosarcoma), and may have a submucosal, subserosal or intraluminal location(Dufresne AC et al; 1999, Buckley JA et al;1998). Malignant stromal tumour of the rectum represents 0.5% of all rectal tumours and 7% of gastrointestinal stromal tumours (GIST)(Wolf O et al;1994, Randleman CD Jr et al;1989). Macroscopically the tumour originates from the muscularis propria of the rectum, and the mucosa generally remains intact. Microscopic findings consist of a proliferation of spindle cells arranged in fascicles(Dufresne AC et al;1999). On endorectal ultrasound, a GIST is seen as a hypoechoic, heterogeneous polycyclical mass, which at high resolution ultrasound imaging is shown to originate from the muscularis propria(Dufresne AC et al; 1999, Marcy PY et al;1993). Endorectal ultrasound is very helpful in defining the extent of disease(Hsieh JS et al;1999). CT appearances of GIST located in the rectum do not differ from those in other parts of the digestive tract. On nonenhanced CT, a GIST presents as a welldelineated, lobulated, homogeneous soft tissue mass with low attenuation and sometimes with calcification(Buckley JA et al;1998, Pannu HK et al; 1999). Although GIST confined to the rectal wall can be treated by local excision(Cailliez-Tomasi JP et al;1999), the prognosis of GIST of the rectum is poor and the 5-year survival rate ranges from 22% to 66% for high grade malignant and low grade malignant types, respectively(Witzigmann H et al;1995). Tumours with mitotic counts higher than 5 per 10 high power fields, and a size larger than 10 cm have an especially significant risk of recurrence(Miettinen M et al,1998).

GIST's of the rectum are most often clinically silent. Symptoms are not specific but highly size-related : the tumors ranged from small asymptomatic intramural nodules to larger masses that bulge into the pelvis, causing compressive symptoms (pain, constipation, occlusion), or rectal bleeding (sudden or occult) together with anemia and urinary symptoms(LI C. F et al;2005). Endoscopy shows a sub-mucosal mass bulging under a normal or ulcerated mucosae. Per-endoscopic guided biopsies can be performed but remained negative in more than 50% of cases(BLAY J. Y et al;2005). Ultra-sonic endoscopy may revealed a hypoechogenic circular lesion with clear edges. Percutaneous needle biopsies have been suggested to be helpful in the diagnosis but may expose to a non-negligible haemorrhage risk and a possible peritoneal diffusion of the tumor(BLAY J. Y et al; 2005).

Timing for surgery is still controversial, although some authors have published indications for surgery(CHANGCHIEN C. R et al;2004): lesions including malignant criteria (Group I), lesions less than 3 cm long with irregular edges and heterogenicity at echoendoscopy screening (Group II). If patients are at high operative risk, periodic biopsies and observation are mandatory. Lesions without malignant criteria (Group III) require echoendoscopy observation every 6 months. lymph node metastasis is considered an infrequent event in the natural evolution of these tumor. Although a limited lymphadenectomy is considered to be the procedure of choice. In this instance, a total mesorectum excision (TME), as strongly recommended for adenocarcinoma, is not mandatory for the resection of rectal GIST. More, extended lymph node dissection doesn't contribute to the improvement of survival(APARICIO T et al;2004).

6. Esophageal GISTs

The presenting signs and symptoms of esophageal GIST depend on the size and location of the tumor. Typically, they cause dysphagia, suggesting the possibility of carcinoma(Miettinen M et al;2000). Less commonly they are detected as large mediastinal masses involving the esophagus. Other manifestations include cough, gastrointestinal bleeding, and weight loss. Occasionally, it may be an incidental finding. There is little information in the literature describing the radiologic appearance of esophageal GISTs. In Miettinen's series, esophageal GISTs ranged from 2.6 to 25 cm in size and were most commonly located in the distal third of the esophagus . This was a distal esophageal mass that distorted and widened the esophageal lumen on barium esophagram(Miettinen M et al;2000). Although complete surgical resection is the standard treatment for localized resectable GISTs, the optimum extent of resection has not been determined. Surgery for esophageal tumors is either enucleation or esophagectomy,with the latter having a higher morbidity rate. Enucleation with clear dissection is sufficient for small-sized,well-capsulated tumors confined to the esophageal muscle layer, without mucosal lesions. Preoperative biopsy and esophagectomy, however, should be considered for larger tumors or tumors accompanied by mucosal lesions. Clear resection margins are also important. In performing enucleation, we shelled out the tumor carefully. with Endo Peanut (U.S. Surgical, Norwalk, CT). And rather than assessing margin status, we determined whether the tumor capsule was maintained in intact condition, as well as confirming mucosal integrity, by intraoperative endoscopic examination. During esophagectomy the external lateral margin as well as the proximal and distal resection margins was confirmed by pathologic examination. Although small intestinal and gastric GISTs may be resected with segmental or wedge resections, esophageal GIST resections are essentially limited to either simple enucleation or esophagectomy. Successful surgical treatment of GISTs depends on complete local resection. The approach to esophagectomy for GISTs should minimize blunt or blind dissection as this will not reliably include maintaining the thin potential barrier of pleura that may overlie extramucosal tumor. Additionally, poor tumor integrity and lack of esophageal serosa increase the risk of tumor rupture with blunt dissection. Transhiatal esophagectomy would likely violate tumors of the distal and midesophagus that extend beyond the muscularis and cannot be recommended. A transthoracic en bloc resection of the pleura overlying the esophagus and any involved surrounding tissues, including diaphragm, is advisable to avoid microscopically or macroscopically incomplete resection. A left thoracoabdominal approach is advocated for larger tumors at the gastroesophageal junction as this will allow excellent visualization of the parahiatal tissue. Management guidelines for GISTs have been defined by consensus of the National Comprehensive Cancer Network (NCCN) and the European Society of Medical Oncology(Demetri GD et al;2006, Blay JY et al;2005). The NCCN guidelines state that enucleation of small (_2 cm) esophageal GIST may be acceptable and that small intraabdominal tumors might be resected laparoscopically.

6.1 Treatment of the non-metastatic disease approach to the primary lesion (extra gastrointestinal tumors and Meckel's diverticulum)

GIST also occur in the extra-intestinal abdominopelvic sites such as the omentum, mesentery, or retroperitoneum. A small number may originate not from the omentum, but from outside the gastrointestinal tract; these are designated extra-GISTs (EGISTs)(Reith JD et al;2000). The reported cases of extra-gastrointestinal stromal tumors (EGIST) have included omental, mesenteric, and retroperitoneal tumors. The cellular origin of GIST from the interstitial cell of Cajal (ICC) raises the question of whether these EGIST are truly an entity analogous to GISTs. It is not well known if extra-gastrointestinal stromal tumors (EGIST) originate from pacemaker cells outside of the GI tract or if mesenchymal cells have the ability to recapitulate the phenotype. Sakurai *et al.*(Sakurai S et al;2001), published their results on the cytological, immunohistochemical, and genetic analysis of 5 omental mesenchymal tumors in 2001. They found all five tumors to be positive for CD117 and CD34 staining, while all were negative for smooth-muscle cell markers. More importantly, the authors reported finding KIT immunoreactive CD117 and CD34 cells within specimens of omentum(Sakurai S et al;2001). These findings and those of Yamamoto *et al.*(Yamamoto H et al;2004) underscore the fact that histologically, EGISTs have a similar appearance to GISTs, and that EGIST is a distinctive entity, different from leiomyosarcomas(Miettinen M et al;1999). The most common mutation of the KIT gene occurred in exon 11 in Sakurai's and Yamamoto's experience(Sakurai S et al;2001, Yamamoto H et al;2004).

GIST arising from Meckel's diverticulum are extremely rare(Johnston AT et al;2001). (Figüre 1,3). The tumors are infrequent and observed only in 0.5–3.2% of the Meckel's diverticula. Of these, 12% tumors are GIST. Radiological appearances of GIST may include asymmetrical thickening of the bowel wall initially, but more commonly an exophytic soft tissue mass with relatively well defined margins is seen(Macari M et al;2001). Areas of necrosis are present in up to 70% of tumours(Nicola´s AI et al;1999) and particularly in larger tumours that frequently undergo central necrosis, due to rapid growth, and subsequent ischaemia (Macari M et al;2001). These also demonstrate heterogeneous contrast enhancement (Macari

M et al; 2001). Areas of calcification and haemorrhage are seen within 7% and 64% of tumours, respectively(Nicola´s AI et al;1999).Surgical resection is the treatment of choice for these tumors, which usually have a poor prognosis. Extragastrointestinal stromal tumors arising in the pancreas are extremely rare. A primary localization in the pancreas has rarely been reported on cytology. The clinical symptoms include abdominal pain, early satiety, flatulence, ileus, bleeding, anemia, and weight loss. It can be diagnosed incidentally by radiologic imaging(Miettinen M;2001). There was a distinct female predominance, age ranging from 38 to 72 years including all surgical pathological cases (mean age 55 years). The majority occurred in the body and tail of the pancreas with an average size of 12 cm(Miettinen M;2001). Extraintestinal gastrointestinal stromal tumors (EGISTs) are uncommon and unique neoplasms, usually involving the mesentery, omentum, retroperitoneum, rarely bladder(Nagase S et al;2007) and inguinal hernial sac. EGISTs arising in the rectovaginal septum and presenting as a recurrent vaginal mass is unusual. The current definitive treatment for EGIST is surgical resection, but in majority of the patients, the tumors recur despite complete resection(Dematteo RP et al;2000). An accurate diagnosis is mandatory for EGIST as these are tumors with an aggressive course and a potential for recurrence inspite of complete surgical excision. In addition, the treatment strategy includes kit tyrosine inhibitor, Imatinib which is used for recurrent and advanced disease.

6.2 Treatment of the metastatic and relapsed disease

GISTs have a high risk of metastatic relapse. The usual site of recurrence is the liver (65%), the peritoneal surface (50%) and both (20%). GIST's response to conventional chemotherapy is very poor (<10%), while radiotherapy is only used for analgesic purposes or in cases of intra peritoneal hemorrhage (Gupta P et al; 2008). Surgery has limited efficacy in the treatment of recurrent and metastatic GIST. In the past years, there has been no efficient method to cure recurrent GIST. GIST is also resistant to both chemotherapy and radiotherapy. The development of imatinib has improved the management of GIST. Even though imatinib is effective for most patients with a metastatic GIST, the development of resistance to the drug is a problem that has been increasing(Heinrich MC;2006). Based on the satisfied result for advanced GIST, surgery combined with imatinib adjuvant therapy may give a hope for the patients with high-risk GISTs. A prospective multicenter trial in high-risk patients after complete gross resection of the tumor revealed that imatinib 400 mg daily can reduce the risk of recurrence and metastasis(Zhan WH et al;2006). Based on the satisfied result for advanced GIST, surgery combined with imatinib adjuvant therapy may give a hope for the patients with high-risk GISTs(Zhan WH et al;2006). Although there are several reports of combination therapy of imatinib with surgery for the advanced GIST with metastases, most of the studies used imatinib eoadjuvantly, and the surgery was performed after the reduction of tumor burden by imatinib therapy. For tumours with a larger diameter and/or unfavourable location, primary wedge resection is often not possible and total or subtotal gastrectomy would be required for resection with tumour-free margins. For these cases, the NCCN guidelines(National Comprehensive Cancer Network (NCCN);2008) and ESMO recommendations(P. G. Casali et al;2008) suggest neoadjuvant imatinib therapy to decrease tumour size, thus fallowing for organ-preserving surgery.

7. Laparoscopic resection

The latest ESMO Clinical Recommendations consider a laparoscopic approach "if cancer surgery principles are respected." (P. G. Casali et al;2008). Current NCCN guidelines do not contain a clear statement on whether surgery for GIST should be performed laparoscopically or through open surgery but recommend that surgery should produce minimal surgical morbidity(National Comprehensive Cancer Network (NCCN);2008). Current recommendation(Guitierrez JC et al;2007) is that laparoscopy should be restricted to the treatment of small lesions (up to 5 cm) due to the possibility of tumor rupture as a result of the manipulation of larger lesions(Guitierrez JC et al;2007). Although oncologic success has been reported with laparoscopic resections(Catena F et al;2008), studies with a larger number of cases and long-term follow-up are required in order to define the actual role of laparoscopy in the treatment of this neoplasm. Laparoscopic surgery as the new "gold standard" in the treatment of localised GISTs of the stomach, it would be highly desirable to have results from one or several randomised controlled trials(S. Sauerland et al;1999). As in other laparoscopic procedures, the existence of a "learning curve"must be assumed and it can be expected that operation times further decrease with growing experience(S.Avital et al;2006, M. Lim et al;2006, R. B. Shin et al,2005).

8. Conclusion

Although rare among tumors involving the gastrointestinal system, gastrointestinal stromal tumors are the most frequent mesenchymal tumors. Recommended treatment regimens need to be updated as the multidisciplinary approach to both diagnosis and treatment of the tumor gains importance. Surgery still holds place as the most important constituent of multidisciplinary in current algorythms and ongoing studies. The introduction of imatinib in clinical practice(Joensuu H et al;2001). changed not only the survival of metastatic GIST patients, but also meant breaking through well established paradigms. Nevertheless, despite the advances and the encouraging outcomes with the use of imatinib, the surgeon still has a key role in the management of GIST(Linhares E et al;2006).

9. References

[1] Abbas M, Farouk Y, Nasr MM, Elsebae MM, Farag A, Akl MM, et al. Gastrointestinal stromal tumors (GISTs): clinical presentation, diagnosis, surgical treatment and its outcome. J Egypt Soc Parasitol 2008;38:883-894.

[2] Aparicio T, Boige V, Sabourin JC et al. Prognostic factors after surgery of primary resectable gastrointestinal stromal tumors. Eur J Surg Oncol 2004;30:1098-1103.

[3] S. Avital, H. Hermon, R. Greenberg, E. Karin, and Y. Skornick, "Learning curve in laparoscopic colorectal surgery: our first 100 patients," *Israel Medical Association Journal*, vol. 8, no. 10, pp. 683–686, 2006.

[4] B. Nilsson, P. B¨umming, J. M. Meis-Kindblom, et al., "Gastrointestinal stromal tumors: the incidence, prevalence, clinical course, and prognostication in the preimatinib mesylate era—a population-based study in western Sweden," *Cancer*, vol. 103, no. 4, pp. 821–829, 2005.

[5] Blay JY, Bonvalot S, Casali P, et al. Consensus, meeting for the management of gastrointestinal stromal tumors: report of the GIST consensus, conference of 20-21 March 2004, under the auspices of ESMO. Ann Onc 2005;16:566–78.

[6] Bucher P, Egger JF, Gervaz P, Ris F, Weintraub D, Villiger P, et al. An audit of surgical management of gastrointestinal stromal tumours (GIST). Eur J Surg Oncol 2006;32:310-314.

[7] Buckley JA, Fishman EK. CT evaluation of small bowel neoplasms: spectrum of disease. Radiographics 1998;18:379-92.

[8] Burkill GJC, Badran M, Thomas JM, Judson IR, Fisher C, Moskovic EC. Malignant Gastrointestinal Stromal Tumour: Distribution, Imaging Features, and Pattern of Metastatic Spread. Radiology 2003;226:527-32.

[9] P. G. Casali, L. Jost, P. Reichardt, M. Schlemmer, and J.- Y. Blay, "Gastrointestinal stromal tumors: ESMO clinical recommendations for diagnosis, treatment and follow-up," *Annals of Oncology*, vol. 19, supplement 2, pp. ii35–ii38, 2008.

[10] Casper ES: Gastrointestinal stromal tumors. *Curr Treat Options Oncol* 2000, 1:267-273

[11] Cailliez-Tomasi JP, Bouche O, Avisse C,Ramaholimihaso F, Diebold MD, Flament JB. Leiomyosarcome du rectum. Quatre nouvelles observations. Gastroenterol Clin Biol 1999;23:523-7.

[12] Catena F, Battista M, Fusaroli P, Ansaloni L, Scioscio V, Santini D et al. Laparoscopic treatment of gastric GIST: report of 21 cases and literature's review. J Gastrointestin Surg. 2008; 12(3):561-8. Epub 2007 Nov 27.

[13] CHANGCHIEN C. R., WU M. C., TASI W. S., CHIANG J. M., CHEN J. S., HUANG S. F., YEH C. Y. Evaluation of prognosis for the malignant rectal gastrointestinal stromal tumor by clinical parameters and immunohistochemical staining. *Dis Colon Rectum*, 2004 Nov, 47 (11) : 1922-9.

[14] Chang MS, Choe G, Kim WH, Kim YI: Small intestinal stromal tumors: a clinicopathologic study of 31 tumors. *Pathol Int* 1998, 48:341-347.

[15] Chen TW, Liu HD, Shyu RY et al. Giant malignant gastrointestinal stromal tumors: recurrence and effects of treatment with STI-571. World J Gastroenterol 2005;11:260-263.

[16] Connolly EM, Gaffney E, Reynolds JV. Gastrointestinal stromal tumors. Br J Surg 2003;90:1178-1186.

[17] Debol SM, Stanley MW, Mallery JS. Can fine needle aspiration cytology adequately diagnose and predict the behavior of gastrointestinal stromal tumors? Adv Anat Pathol. 2001; 8: 93-97.

[18] DeMatteo RP, Lewis JJ, Leung D, Mudan SS, Woodruff JM, Brennan MF: Two hundred gastrointestinal stromal tumors: recurrence patterns and prognostic factors for survival. *Ann Surg* 2000, 231:51-58.

[19] Demetri GD, Baker LH, Benjamin R, et al. DNCCN, soft tissue sarcoma. Clinical practice guidelines in oncology. National Comprehensive Cancer Network; 2006:v.3.

[20] Demetri GD, von Mehren M, Blanke CD, Abbeele AD, Eisenberg B, Roberts PJ, Heinrich MC, Tuveson DA, Singer S, Janicek M, Fletcher JA, Silverman SG, Silberman SL, Capdeville R, Kiese B, Peng B, Dimitrijevic S, Druker BJ, Corless C, Fletcher CD, Joensuu H: Efficacy and safety of imatinib mesylate in advanced gastrointestinal stromal tumors. *N Engl J Med* 2002, 347:472-80.

[21] Dufresne AC, Brocheriou-Spelle I, Boudiaf M, Soyer Ph, Pelage JP, Rymer R. Tumeur stromale maligne rectale (leiomyosarcome): aspects echoendoscopique, tomodensitometrique et correlation anatomopathologique. J Radiol 1999;80: 303-5.
[22] Efremidou EI, Liratzopoulos N, Papageorgiou MS, Romanidis K. Perforated GIST of the small intestine as a rare cause of acute abdomen: Surgical treatment and adjuvant therapy. Case report. J Gastrointestin Liver Dis 2006;15:297-299.
[23] Emory TS, Sobin LH, Lukes L, Lee DH, O'Leary TJ. Prognosis of gastrointestinal smooth-muscle (stromal) tumors. Dependence on anatomic site. Am J Surg Pathol 1999;23:82–7.
[24] C. D. M. Fletcher, J. J. Berman, C. Corless, et al., "Diagnosis of gastrointestinal stromal tumors: a consensus approach,"*Human Pathology*, vol. 33, no. 5, pp. 459–465, 2002.
[25] Fang SH, Dong DJ, Zhang SZ, Jin M. Angiographic findings of gastrointestinal stromal tumor. World J Gastroenterol 2004;10:2905-2907.
[26] Gupta P, Tewari M, Shulka H: Gastrointestinal stromal tumor. *Surg Oncol* 2008, 17(2):129-138.
[27] Gelibter A, Milella M, Ceribelli A et al. PET scanning evaluation of response to imatinib mesylate therapy in gastrointestinal stromal tumor (GIST) patients. Anticancer Res 2004;24:3147- 3151.
[28] Gold JS, De Matteo RP: Combined surgical and molecular therapy: the gastrointestinal stromal tumor model. *Annals of Surgery* 2006, 244:176-184.
[29] Graadt van Roggen JF, van Veithuysen MLF, Hogendoorn PCW. The histopathological differential diagnosis of gastrointestinal tumors. J Clin Pathol 2001;54:96-102.
[30] Guitierrez JC, Oliveira LO, Perez EA, Rocha-Lima C, Livingstone AS, Koniaris LG. Optimizing diagnosis, staging, and management of gastrointestinal stromal tumors. J Am Coll Surg. 2007; 205(3):479-91 (Quiz 524). Epub 2007 Jul 16.
[31] Heinrich MC. Molecular basis for treatment of gastrointestinal stromal tumours. Eur J Cancer. 2006; 4(3 Suppl 1):S10-8.
[32] Hsieh JS, Huang CJ, Wang JY, Huang TJ. Benefits of endorectal ultrasound for management of smooth-muscle tumor of the rectum: report of three cases. Dis Colon Rectum 1999;42:1085-8.
[33] Joensuu H, Roberts PJ, Sarlomo-Rikala M, Anderson LC, Tervahartiala P, Tuveson D, et al. Effect of tyrosine kinase inhibitor STI571 in a patient with a metastatic gastrointestinal stromal tumor. N Engl J Med. 2001; 344(14):1052-6.
[34] Johnston AT, Khan A, Bleakney R, Keenan RA: Stromal tumor within a Meckel's diverticulum: CT and ultrasound findings. *Br J Radiol* 2001, 74:1142-1144.
[35] H. Joensuu, C. Fletcher, S. Dimitrijevic, S. Silberman, P. Roberts, and G. Demetri, "Management of malignant gastrointestinal stromal tumours," *The Lancet Oncology*, vol. 3, no. 11, pp. 655–664, 2002.
[36] G. Kaehler, R. Grobholz, C. Langner, K. Suchan, and S. Post, "A new technique of endoscopic full-thickness resection using a flexible stapler," *Endoscopy*, vol. 38, no. 1, pp. 86–89, 2006.
[37] Karagülle E, Türk E, Yildirim E, Göktürk HS, Kiyici H, Moray G. Multifocal intestinal stromal tumors with jejunal perforation and intra-abdominal abscess: report of a case. Turk J Gastroenterol 2008;19:264-267.

[38] LI C. F., CHUANG S. S., LU C. L., LIN C. N. Gastrointestinal stromal tumor (GIST) in southern Taiwan : a clinicopathologic study of 93 resected cases. *Pathol Res Pract*, 2005, 201 (1) : 1-9.
[39] M. Lim, C. J. O'Boyle, C. M. S. Royston, and P. C. Sedman, "Day case laparoscopic herniorraphy: a NICE procedure with a long learning curve," *Surgical Endoscopy*, vol. 20, no. 9, pp. 1453–1459, 2006.
[40] Linhares E, Valadão M. Atualização em GIST. Rev Col Bras Cir. 2006; 33(1):51-4.
[41] Ludwig DJ, Traverso W. GI stromal tumors and their clinical behaviour. Am J Surg 1997;173:390-4.
[42] Macari M, Balthazar EJ. CT of bowel wall thickening: significance and pitfalls of interpretation. AJR 2001;176:1105–16.
[43] Marcy PY, Francois E, Bruneton JN, Peroux JL, Balu-Maestro C, Melia P, et al. Leiomyosarcome gastrique, echoendoscopie et IRM. J Radiol 1993; 74:583-8.
[44] Miettinen et al 2005 Miettinen M, Sobin LH, Lasota J. 2005. Gastrointestinal stromal tumors of the stomach: a clinicopathologic, immunohistochemical, and molecular genetic study of 1765 cases with long-term follow-up. *Am J Surg Pathol*, 29:52–68.
[45] Miettinen M, Lasota J. Gastrointestinal stromal tumors: pathology and prognosis at different sites. Semin Diagn Pathol 2006;23:70-83.
[46] Miettinen M, Monihan JM, Sarlomo-Rikala M, Kovatich AJ, Carr NJ, Emory TS, Sobin LH: Gastrointestinal stromal tumors/smooth muscle tumors (GISTs) primary in the omentum and mesentery: clinicopathologic and immunohistochemical study of 26 cases. *Am J Surg Pathol* 1999, 23:1109-1118.
[47] Miettien M, Sarlomo-Rikala M, Sobin LH, Lasota J. Gastrointestinal stromal tumors and leiomyosarcomas in the colon. Am J Surg Path 2000;24:1339-52.
[48] Miettinen M, Sarlomo-Rikala M, Sobin LH, Lasota J. Esophageal stromal tumors: a clinicopathologic, immunohistochemical, and molecular genetic study of 17 cases and comparison with esophageal leiomyomas and leiomyosarcomas. Am J Surg Pathol 2000; 24: 211-222.
[49] Miettinen M, Sarlomo-Rikala M, Lasota J. Gastrointestinal stromal tumours. Ann Chir Gynaecol 1998;87:278-81.
[50] Miettinen M. Are desmoid tumors kit positive? Am J Surg Pathol 2001; 25:549-50.
[51] Mukhopadyay S, Gupta SD. Gastrointestinal Stromal Tumours : Bench-to-bedside review. GI Surgery Annual 2002;9:101-48.
[52] Nagase S, Mikami Y, Moriya T, Niikura H, Yoshinaga K, Takano T. Vaginal tumors with histologic and immunocytochemical feature of gastrointestinal stromal tumor: two cases and review of the literature. Int J Gynecol Cancer. 2007 Jul-Aug; 17(4): 928-33.
[53] National Comprehensive Cancer Network (NCCN), "Practice Guidelines in Oncology, v.2.2008," 2008.
[54] Nakagohri T, Kenmochi T, Kainuma O, Tokoro Y, Kobayashi S, Asano T. Inferior head resection of the pancreas for intraductal papillary mucinous tumors. Am J Surg 2000;179:482–4.
[55] Nicola´s AI, Elduayen B, Vivas I, Paniz A, Martinez SHY, Cuesta A, et al. Radiological appearances of gastrointestinal stromal tumours. In: European Congress of Radiology; 1999 March7–12; Vienna, Austria. European Congress of Radiology, 1999.

[56] Novitsky YW, Kercher KW, Sing RF, et al. 2006. Long-term outcomes of laparoscopic resection of gastric gastrointestinal stromal tumors. *Ann Surg*, 243:738–45; discussion 745–7.

[57] Ng EH, Pollock RE, Munsell MF, Atkinson EN, Romsdahl MM: Prognostic factors influencing survival in gastrointestinal leiomyosarcomaImplications for surgical management and staging. *Ann Surg* 1992, 215:68-77.

[58] Pannu HK, Hruban R, Fishman EK. CT of gastric leiomyosarcoma: patterns of involvement. AJR 1999;173:369-73.

[59] Pidhorechly I, Cheney RT, Lraybill WG, Gibbs JF. Gastrointestinal stromal tumors: Current diagnosis, biologic behavior, and management. Ann Surg Oncol 2000;7:705–12.

[60] Pieri JPEN, Choudry U, Muzikansky A, Yeap BY, Souba WW, Ott MJ. The effect of surgery and grade on outcome of gastrointestinal stromal tumors. Arch Surg 2001;136:383–9.

[61] Randleman CD Jr, Wolff BG, Dozois RR, Spencer RJ, Weiland LH, Ilstrup DM. Leiomyosarcoma of the rectum and anus: a series of 22 cases. Int J Colorectal Dis 1989;4:91-6.

[62] Reith JD, Goldblum JR, Lyles RH, Weiss SW: Extragastrointestinal (soft tissue) stromal tumors: an analysis of 48 cases with emphasis on histologic predictors of outcome. *Mod Pathol* 2000,13((5)):577-585.

[63] Roberto Logrono , Dennie Jones V, Sohaib Faruqi , Manoop Bhutani S: Recent advances in cell biology, diagnosis and therapy of gastrointestinal stromal tumor (GIST). *Cancer Biology and Therapy* 2004, 33:251-258.

[64] Roberts PJ, Eisenberg B: Clinical presentation of gastrointestinal stromal tumors and treatment of operable disease. *Eur J Cancer* 2002, 38:S37-38.

[65] Rutkowski et al 2007 Rutkowski P, Nowecki ZI, Michej W, et al. 2007. Risk criteria and prognostic factors for predicting recurrences after resection of primary gastrointestinal stromal tumor. *Ann Surg Oncol*, 14:2018–27.

[66] S. Sauerland, R. Lefering, and E. A. M. Neugebauer, "The pros and cons of evidence-based surgery," *Langenbeck's Archives of Surgery*, vol. 384, no. 5, pp. 423–431, 1999.

[67] S. Singer, B. P. Rubin, M. L. Lux, et al., "Prognostic value ofKIT mutation type, mitotic activity, and histologic subtype ingastrointestinal stromal tumors," *Journal of Clinical Oncology*,vol. 20, no. 18, pp. 3898–3905, 2002.

[68] R. B. Shin, "Evaluation of the learning curve for laparoscopic Roux-en-Y gastric bypass surgery," *Surgery for Obesity and Related Diseases*, vol. 1, no. 2, pp. 91–94, 2005.

[69] Shiu MH, Farr GH, Papchristou DN, Hajdu SI: Myosarcoma of the stomach: nature history, prognostic factors and management. *Cancer* 1982, 49:177-187.

[70] Spinelli GP, Miele E, Tomao F, Rossi L, Pasciuti G, Zullo A, Zoratto F, Nunnari J, Pisanelli GC, Tomao S. The synchronous occurrence of squamous cell carcinoma and gastrointestinal stromal tumor (GIST) at esophageal site. *World J Surg Oncol* 2008; 6: 116.

[71] Spivach A, Zanconati F, Bonifacio Gori D, Pellegrino M, Sinconi A. Stromal tumors of the small intestine (GIST). Prognostic differences based on clinical, morphological and immunophenotypic features. Minerva Chir. 1999;54:717-724.

[72] Sakamoto Y, Nagai M, Tanaka N, Nobori M, Tsukamoto T, Nokubi M, et al. Anatomical segmentectomy of the head of the pancreas along the embryologically fusion-plane: A feasible procedure? Surgery 2000;128: 822–31.
[73] Sakamoto Y, Tanaka N, Nagai M, Nobori M, Otani T, Makuuchi M. Anterior segmentectomy of the pancreatic head for islet cell tumors. Pancreas 2002;24:317–9.
[74] Sakurai S, Hishima T, Takazawa Y, Sano T, Nakajima T, Saito K, Morinaga S, Fukayama M: Gastrointestinal stromal tumors and KIT-positive mesenchymal cells in the omentum. *Pathol Int* 2001, 51:524-531.
[75] Sturgeon C, Chejfec G, Espat NJ: Gastrointestinal stromal tumors: a spectrum of disease. *Surg Oncol* 2003, 12:21-26.
[76] Tashiro T, Hasegawa T, Omatsu M, Sekine S, Shimoda T, Katai H:Gastrointestinal stromal tumor of the stomach showing lymph node metastases. *Histopathology* 2005, 47:438-439.
[77] Thayer SP, Fernandez-del Castillo C, Balcom JH, Warshaw AL. Complete dorsal pancreatectomy with preservation of the ventral pancreas: a new surgical technique. Surgery 2002;131:577–80.
[78] Tran T, Davila JA, El-Serag HB. The epidemiology of malignant gastrointestinal stromal tumors: an analysis of 1,458 cases from 1992 to 2000. Am J Gastroenterol. 2005; 100: 162-168.
[79] Tworedk JA, Appelman HD, Singleton TP, Greenson JK: Stromal tumors of the jejunum and ileum. *Mod Pathol* 1997, 10:200-209.
[80] Uehara K, Hasegawa H, Ogiso S, Sakamoto E, Shibahara H, Igami T, et al. Gastrointestinal stromal tumor of the duodenum: Diagnosis and treatment. Geka 2001;63:1058–61 (in Japanese).
[81] Van Der Zwan SM, Dematteo RP. 2005. Gastrointestinal stromal tumor: 5 years later. *Cancer*, 104:1781–8.
[82] Vander Noot MR 3rd, Eloubeidi MA, Chen VK et al. Diagnosis of gastrointestinal tract lesions by endoscopic ultrasound-guided fine-needle aspiration biopsy. Cancer 2004;102:157-163.
[83] Winfield , Robert D, Hochwald , Steven N, Vogel , Stephen B, Hemming , Alan W, Liu , Chen , Cance , William G, Grobmyer , Stephen R: *American Surgeon*. 2006, 72:719-23.
[84] Witzigmann H, Sagasser J, Leipprandt E, Witte J. Leiomyosarcoma of the rectum. Zentralbl Chir 1995;120:69-72.
[85] Wolf O, Glaser F, Kuntz C, Lehnert T. Endorectal ultrasound and leiomyosarcoma of the rectum. Clin Investig 1994;72:381-4.
[86] Yamamoto H, Oda Y, Kawaguchi K, Nakamura N, Takahira T, Tamiya S, Saito T, Oshiro Y, Ohta M, Yao T, Tsuneyoshi M: c-kit and PDGFRA mutations in extragastrointestinal stromal tumor (gastrointestinal stromal tumor of the soft tissue). *Am J Surg Pathol* 2004, 28:479-488.
[87] Zhan WH, Wang PZ, Shao YF, Wu XT, Gu J, Li R, et al. Efficacy and safety of adjuvant post-surgical therapy with imatinib in gastrointestinal stromal tumor patients with high risk of recurrence: interim analysis from a multicenter prospective clinical trial. Chin J Gastrointest Surg (Chin) 2006; 9: 383-387.

[88] Yamamoto H, Oda Y, Kawaguchi K, Nakamura N, Takahira T, Tamiya S, Saito T, Oshiro Y, Ohta M, Yao T, Tsuneyoshi M: c-kit and PDGFRA mutations in extragastrointestinal stromal tumor (gastrointestinal stromal tumor of the soft tissue). *Am J Surg Pathol* 2004, 28:479-488.

[89] Y. Shinomura, K. Kinoshita, S. Tsutsui, and S. Hirota, "Pathophysiology, diagnosis, and treatment of gastrointestinal stromal tumors," *Journal of Gastroenterology*, vol. 40, no. 8, pp. 775–780, 2005.

6

Gastrointestinal Stromal Tumor of the Rectovaginal Septum, a Diagnosis Challenge

Josefa Marcos Sanmartín, María José Román Sánchez, José Antonio López Fernández, Óscar Piñero Sánchez, Amparo Candela Hidalgo, Hortensia Ballester Galiana, Natalia Esteve Fuster, Aránzazu Saco López and Juan Carlos Martínez Escoriza
Department of Gynaecology, Hospital General Universitario, Alicante Spain

1. Introduction

Gastrointestinal stromal tumors (GISTs) are the most common mesenchymal tumors of the gastrointestinal tract. These are rare tumors representing approximately 0.1-3.0% of all gastrointestinal cancers and approximately 5% of all soft tissue sarcomas (Reid et al., 2005; Fletcher et al., 2002). Due to their similar appearance by light microscopy, GISTs were previously thought to be smooth muscle neoplasms, and most were classified as leiomyosarcoma (Reid et al, 2005). (Table 1) The precise cellular origin of these tumors has been proposed to be the interstitial cell of Cajal, an interstitial pacemaker cell (Connolly et al., 2003).

It is important to differentiate between GISTs, which constitute approximately 80% of gastrointestinal mesenchymal tumors, and the less common gastrointestinal non-epithelial neoplasms, leiomyoma, leiomyosarcoma (10-15% of mesenchymal tumors), schwannomas (5%), and other malignant disorders.

Nearly all GISTs (90-100%) display strong immunohistochemical staining for *kit* (CD 117), and this can be used in their differential diagnosis and positive identification. Smooth muscle neoplasms, and neurogenic tumours (schwannoma) typically do not show a positive expression of CD117, but can be distinguished from GISTs by histological and clinical means. It is recommended that CD117 immunostaining should be performed to facilitate the diagnosis of GISTs for spindle cell or epithelioid tumors arising the gastrointestinal tract. Diagnosis, however, should not be based purely on CD117 expression. The diagnosis of CD117 negative GISTs should only be made with extreme care. If there is evidence of desmin or S-100 expression and the tumor is not associated with the gut wall then a diagnosis of a *kit* negative GIST should not be made.

Mutations of *kit* are common in malignant GISTs and lead to constitutional activation of tyrosine kinase function, which causes cellular proliferation and resistance to apoptosis. It is also important the stain for the myeloid stem cell antigen CD 34 in 53% to 71% of cases. (Connolly et al., 2003; De Matteo et al., 2000; Saund et al., 2004, Yamamoto et al., 2004).

	CD 117	CD 34	SMA	Desmin	S-100
GIST	+ Around 95%	+ 60-70%	+ 30-40%	Very rare	+ 5%
Smooth Muscle Tumor	-	+ 10-15%	+	+	Rare
Schwannoma	-	+	-	-	+

Table 1. Immunohistochemical schema for the differential diagnosis of spindle cell tumors of the gastrointestinal tract. (Reid et al., 2005).

Approximately, 30% of GISTs are malignant. The principal sites of metastasis are the liver and the peritoneal cavity. Rarely, GISTs metastasise to other sites such as the lymph nodes, lung, bone (Reid et al., 2005), and muscle (Pasku et al., 2008).
The most frequent anatomic sites of tumor origin are the stomach (70%), the small intestine (20-30%), esophagus, colon and rectum (10%) (Reid et al., 2005). (Table 2).

Site	**Percentage**
Stomach	60-70%
Small intestine	20-30%
Oesophagus, mesentery, omentum, colon and rectum	10%

Table 2. Site of GISTs. (Reid et al., 2005)

They are rare before the age of 40 years and very rare in children, with a median age of 50-60 years. Some data show a slight male predominance. (Reid et al., 2005).
The symptoms (Table 3) (Nickl et al., 2004; Reid et al., 2005, Saund et al., 2004) of GISTs are non-especific and depend on the size and location of the lesion. Small GISTs (2cm or less) are usually asymptomatic and are detected during investigations or surgical procedures of unrelated causes. The vast majority of these are low-risk for malignancy. The most common symptom is gastrointestinal bleeding which is present in approximately 50% of patients. Systemic symptoms such as fever, night sweats, and weight loss are common in GISTs and very rare in other sarcomas. Patients with larger tumors may experience abdominal discomfort or develop a palpable mass. Up to 25% of patients present with acute haemorrhage into the intestinal tract or peritoneal cavity from tumor rupture. Symptomatic oesophageal GISTs typically present with dysphagia, while gastric and small intestinal GISTs often present with vage symptoms leading to their eventual detection by gastroscopy or radiology. Most duodenal GISTs occur in the second part of the duodenum where they push or infiltrate into the pancreas. Colorectal GISTs may manifest with pain and gastrointestinal obstruction, and lower intestinal bleeding. Rectal tumors are usually deep intramural tumors.

Symptoms	**Incidence**
Abdominal pain	20-50%
Gastrointestinal bleeeding	50%
Gastrointestinal obstruction	10-30%
Asymptomatic	20%

Table 3. Symptoms of GIST at diagnosis. (Reid et al., 2005)

The pathogenesis of GISTs has been established by the observation that *kit* is highly expressed and mutated in almost all tumors (Taniguchi et al., 1999). The use of antibodies to *kit*, as part of an immunohistochemical panel and in combination with traditional histological and clinical examinations, means that it is possible to distinguish clearly GISTs from other gastrointestinal tract tumours. In addition, the tyrosine kinase inhibitor *imatinib mesilate (Gleevec™)* represents a major breakthrough in the treatment of GISTs, as it has significant antitumour activity in these neoplasms, which are generally resistant to cytotoxic chemotherapy (Zalupski et al. 1991; Ronellenfitsch et al., 2008). A second targeted tyrosine kinase inhibitor, *sunitinib malate (Sutent™)*, has been approved for the treatment of imatinib-resistant gastrointestinal stromal tumors. (Raut et al., 2007).
Surgical resection is the principal treatment for GISTs. Evaluation of the resecability of a GIST is determined by the surgeon and depends on the stage and the individual patient's fitness for surgery. The primary goal of surgery is complete resection of the disease with avoidance of tumor rupture. Care is necessary as GISTs are often soft and fragile, and tumor rupture may seed implants in the peritonel cavity and liver. A wide local resection with macroscopic removal of the entire tumor to achieve microscopic clearance is recommended. An adequate cancer margin is considered to be 2cm (Reid et al.,2005) but this is not always possible.
It is recommended that all patients should be followed up. Observation is the current standard of care after complete resection of a primary tumor. Following initial assessment, high risk tumors should have computed tomography (CT) every 6 months for 3 years. However, in all cases, if symptoms become evident an early CT may be appropriate. Regardless of risk, clinic review should be indefinite, as these tumors may recur several years after apparently curative resection.
There was no currently accepted adjuvant therapy regimen before *Gleevec™* was approved. *Gleevec™* is generally well tolerated at doses up to 800mg/day. Toxicities include nausea and vomiting, diarrhoea, myalgia, skin rash and occasional neutropenia (Table 4). Although frequent, these toxicities rarely require withdrawal of *Gleevec™*.

Blood and lymphatic system disorders	Neutropenia, thrombocytopenia, anaemia
Nervous system disorders	Headache
Gastrointestinal disorders	Nausea, vomiting, diarrhoea, dyspepsia, abdominal pain
Skin and subcutaneous tissue disorders	Periorbital oedema, dermatitis /eczema /rash
Musculoskeletal, connective tissue and bone disorders	Muscle spam and cramps, musculoskeletal pain including arthralgia
General disorders and Administration site conditions	Fluid retention and oedema, fatigue

Table 4. Very common (>1/10) adverse reactions with *imatinib mesylate* (Reid et al., 2005)

2. Gastrointestinal stromal tumours of the rectovaginal septum

GISTs located out of the gastrointestinal tract (Extragastrointestinal stromal tumors, EGISTs) are very uncommon; and those that arise in the rectovaginal septum are highly infrequent entities, that pose a challenge due to the lack of diagnostic suspicious (Ceballos et al., 2004;

Hellan et al., 2006; Lam et al., 2006; Marcos et al., 2010; Mussi et al., 2008; Nagase et al., 2007; Nasu et al., 2004; Takano et al., 2006; Tooru et al., 2001; Valera et al., 2008; Weppler et al., 2005; Zang et al., 2009).

The main differential diagnosis of EGISTs of the vagina and rectovaginal septum is leiomyoma and leiomyosarcoma. Like GISts, both leiomyoma and leiomyosarcoma are rare primary lesions of the vagina. Histologically, leiomyomas and leiomyosarcomas are usually composed of spindle cells that are arranged in fascicles. In contrast to GISTs, which have very fibrillary, pale pink cytoplasm, smooth muscle tumors have dense, brightly eosinophilic cytoplasm. In addition, leiomyosarcomas tend to exhibit pleomorphism, which is unusual in GIST; smooth muscle tumors are immunoreactive for smooth muscle actin and desmin and are negative for *kit* (CD117). Like GISTs, smooth muscle tumors can be positive for CD34. Epithelioid smooth muscle tumors can mimic both epithelioid GIST and carcinoma, which are the most likely soft tissue neoplasm to arise in this location. Carcinomas are usually strongly positive for cytokeratins, whereas GISTs rarely express this antigen. Nerve sheath tumors, especially schwannomas are diffusely and strongly positive for S-100 protein and negative for *kit*. Aggressive angiomyxoma is rare but tends to occur in the deep soft tissues of the vulva and vagina. In contrast to GIST, these lesions are always paucicellular, contain myxoid stroma and a prominent vascular pattern, are positive for actine, desmin, estrogen receptor, and progesterone receptor, and negative for *kit*. Angiomyofibroblastoma is another spindle cell lesion that enters into the differential diagnosis. They are typically located in the superficial soft tissues and are variably cellular with a prominent vascular pattern. They are negative for *kit* and positive for actin, desmin, estrogen receptor and progesterone receptor. Also, dermatofibrosarcoma protuberans can arise in the vulvovaginal region; they are uniformly positive for CD34, but can be distinguished from GIST because are negative for *kit*.

Because of their malignant potential and recent advances in the management of GISTs with *imatinib mesylate (Gleevec™)* (De Matteo et al., 2007; Park et al., 2008; Verma et al., 2009), it is imperative that these tumors are diagnosed correctly despite of the similarity in their structure and size. Conventional radiotherapy and chemotrapy are useless in the treatment of these tumors, thus this fact makes more important the misdiagnosis of these masses.

However, the current definitive treatment for GIST, including EGIST, is surgical.

In this chapter, we describe a recent case of EGIST located in the rectovaginal septum, and a rewiev of the recent literature in this field.

2.1 Case report

We report the case of a 75-year-old woman with a GIST tumor in the rectovaginal septum. She consulted because of unpleasant feelings in the vagina and constipation that had started few months ago. Colonoscopy (Fig. 1.) revealed a probably submucosal tumor of 4cm in the anterior wall of the lower rectum, but it could not confirm the origin (gynecological or gastrointestinal). The patient was admitted in our Department for close examination and eventual treatment.

During the physical examination we saw a tumour of about 5 cm that stunned in the posterior wall of the vagina; pelvic exmination revealed (Fig. 2.) a 5cm hard, well-circumscribed heterogeneous tumor, with a clear border in the rectovaginal space.

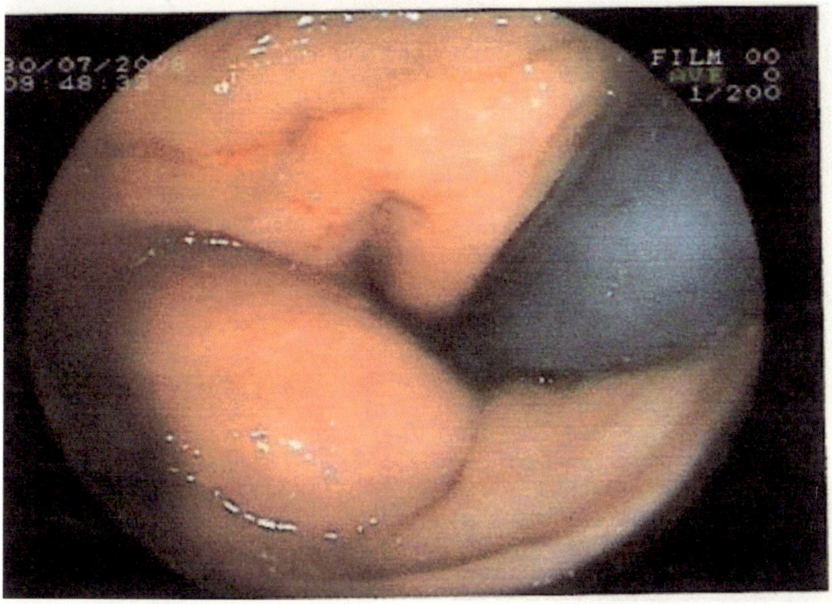

Fig. 1. Colonoscopy: Probably submucosal tumor of 4cm in the anterior wall of the lower rectum.

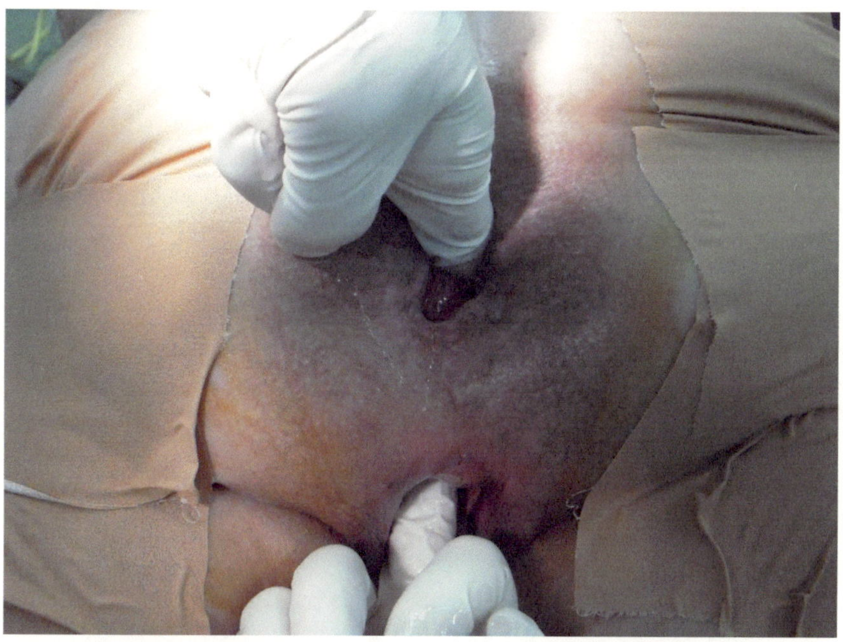

Fig. 2. Pelvic examination revealed a mass between rectum and vagina.

The transvaginal ultrasound showed a normal atrophic internal genitalia; and a tumor well-delimited of about 4-5 cm; the mass appearance was solid with high vascularization. Nuclear magnetic resonance imaging (NMRI) from the abdomen and pelvis was performed, and it showed (Fig. 3, 4 and 5.) the origin of the tumor in the anterior wall of the lower rectum. Tumor markers as carcinoembryonic antigen (CEA), alpha-fetoprotein (AFP) and CA 19.9 were negative.

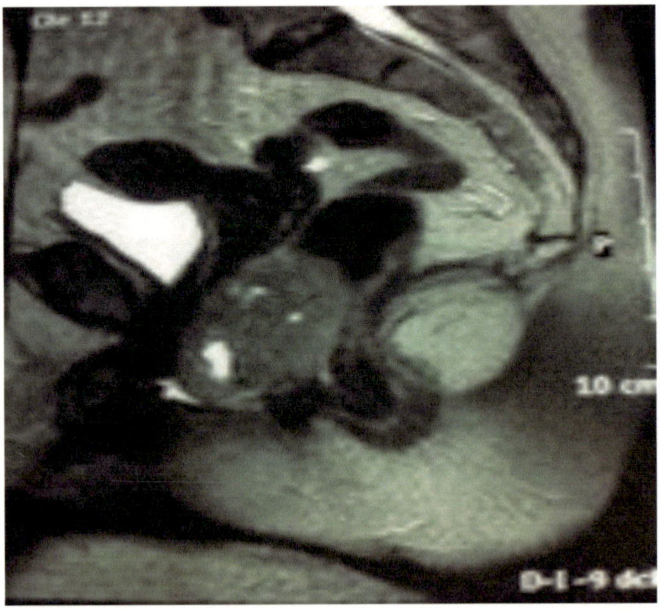

Fig. 3. NMRI that shows the probably origin of the tumor in the anterior wall of the lower rectum.

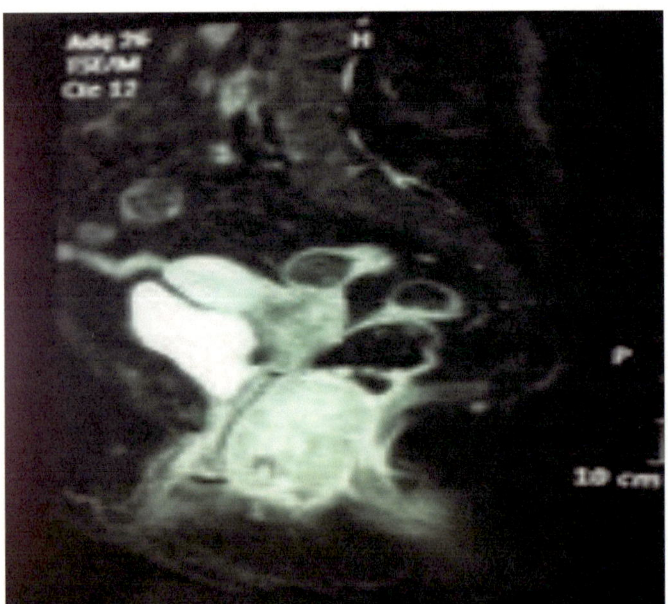

Fig. 4. Another image of NMRI that shows the location of the mass.

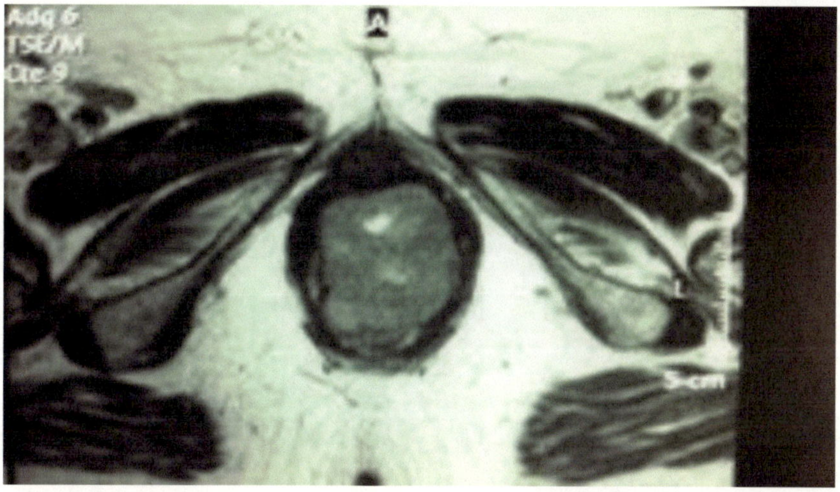

Fig. 5. A transversal section image of NMRI. It shows the mass between vagina and rectum.

Transvaginal biopsy was performed and the specimen was histologically diagnosed as gastrointestinal stromal tumour (c-Kit +) of intermediate risk of malignancy.

A transvaginal tumor enucleation was performed with the colaboration of the Department of Surgery, and also perineal reconstruction was done (Fig. 6, 7, 8 and 9).

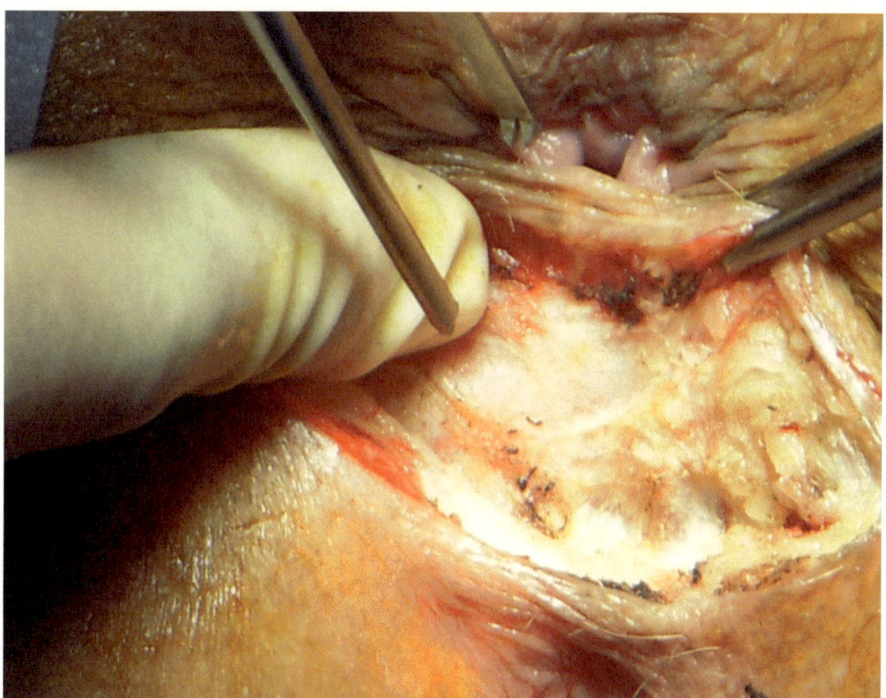

Fig. 6. A transvaginal excision of the tumor was performed.

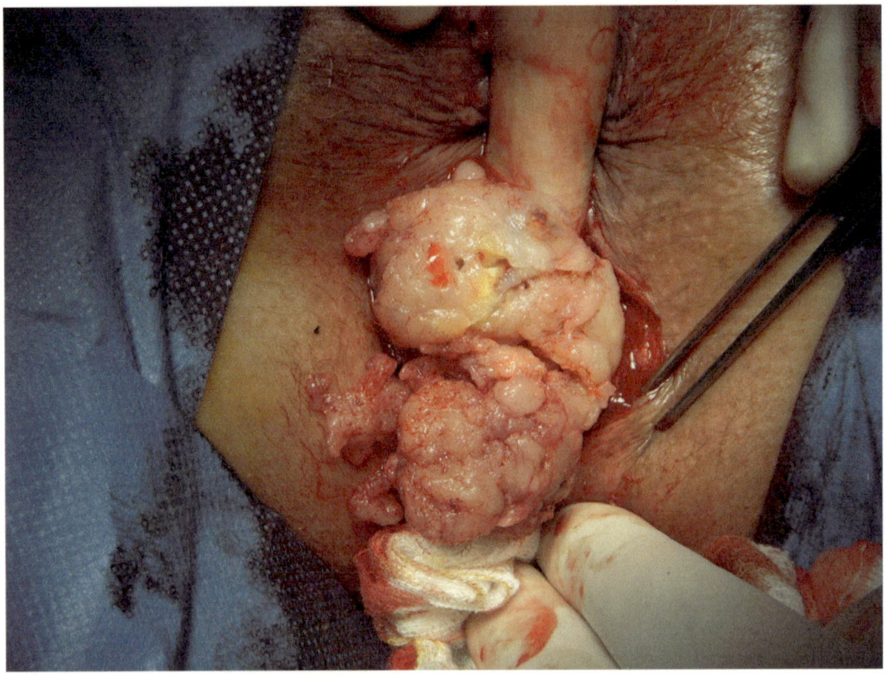

Fig. 7. The tumor was fragile and ruptured during the operation.

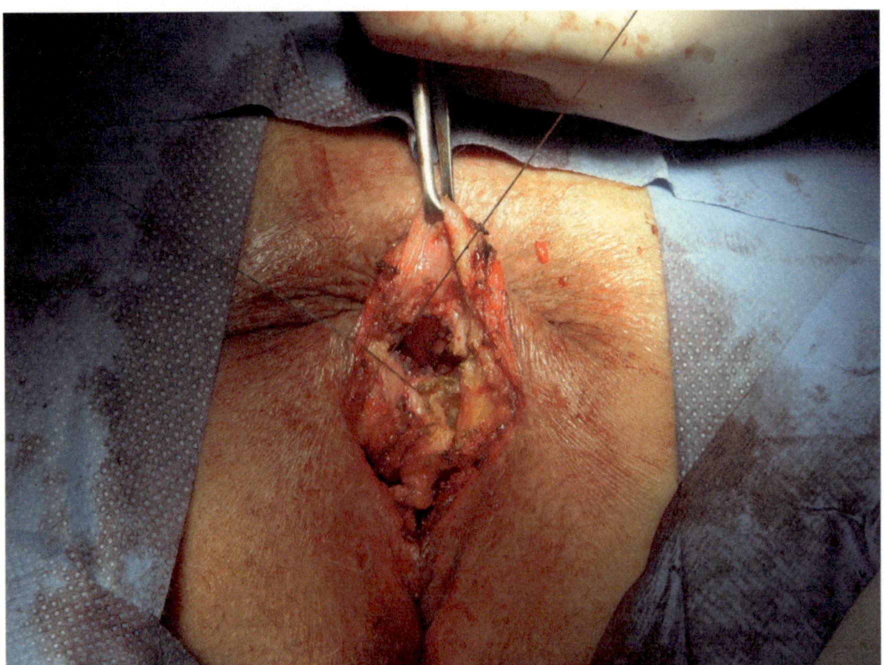

Fig. 8. A perineal reconstruction was also done.

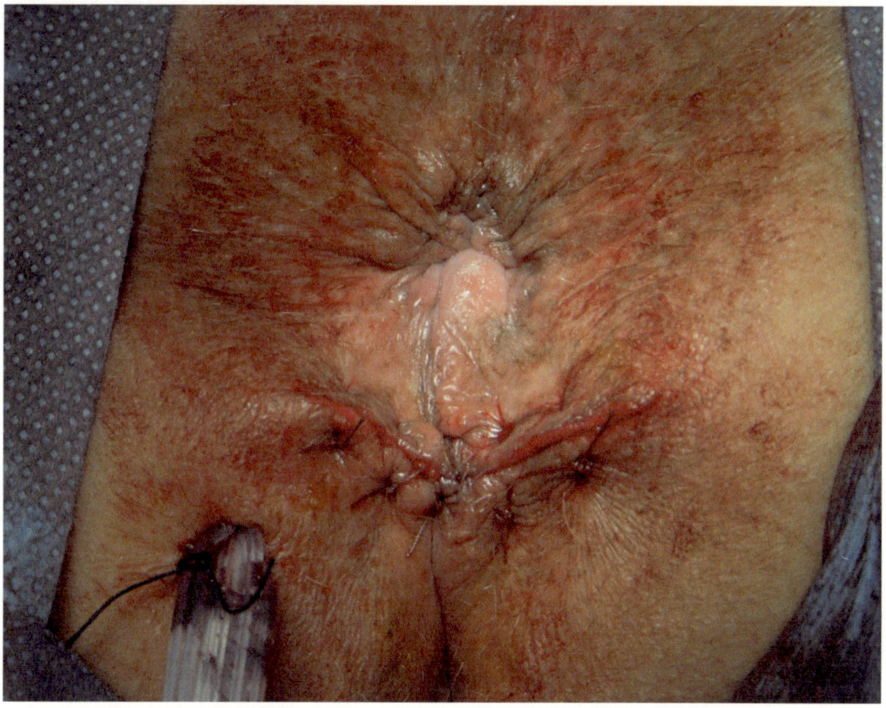

Fig. 9. Final result of the surgery.

The final histological study revealed a gastrointestinal stromal tumour of high risk of malignancy (Fig. 10, 11 and 12) (16 mitotic figures per 50 high power fields, HPF), composed of fascicles of spindle cells with elongated nuclei, fine chromatin, and abundant pale pink, fibrillary cytoplasm. Tumor size and margins could not be evaluated because it had been fragmented during the surgical excision, so because of the high probability of an incomplete

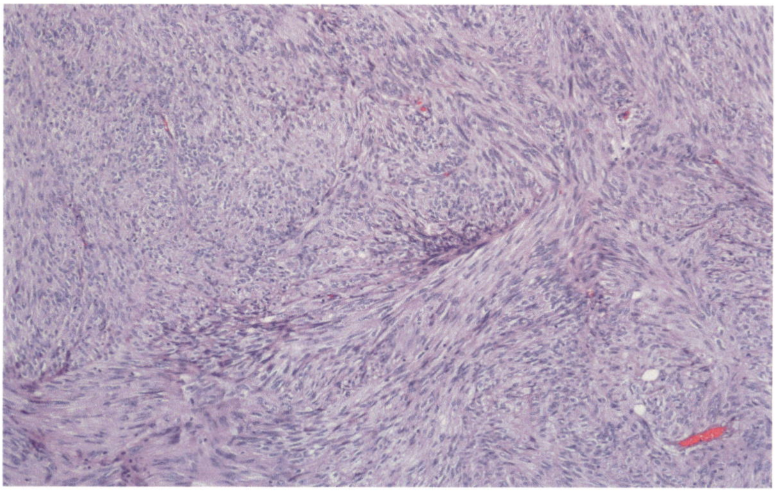

Fig. 10. Fascicles of spindle cells with elongated nuclei, fine chromatin, and abundant pale pink, fibrillary cytoplasm.

surgey, adyuvant treatment with *imatinib mesylate* was established without important toxicity (*Gleevec*™, 400mg per day in an oral dose). After one year following this treatment, the patient was disease free and now, 3 years later, is following rutinary controls with no evidence of disease.

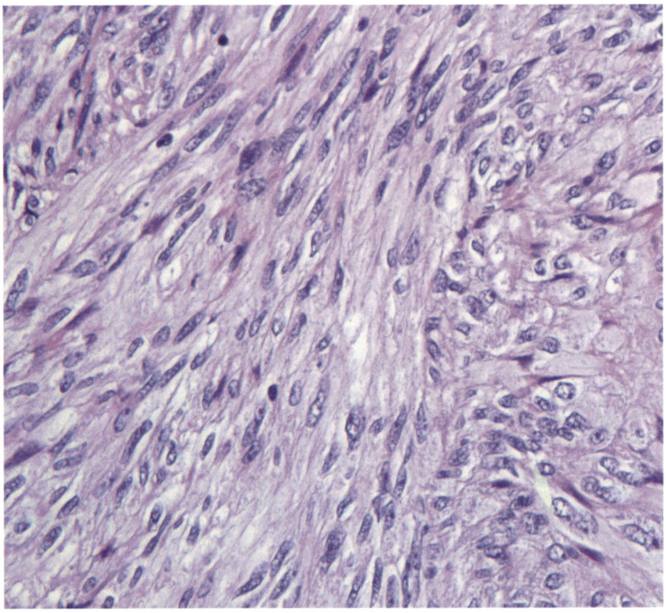

Fig. 11. Original magnification, x 400.

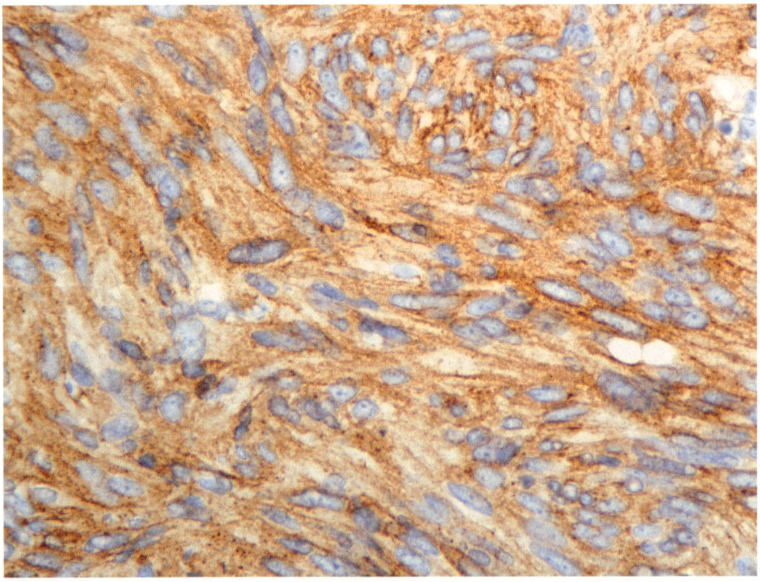

Fig. 12. Inmunohistochemical finding of the tumor cells. Tumor cells show strong and diffuse positivity for immunoreactive *c-kit* (original magnificaction, x 400)

2.2 Discussion

EGISTs comprises about 5-7% of all GISTs. The majority of them have involved the mesentery, omentum, and retroperitoneum. Only eleven cases of them presenting as a vaginal mass have been reported previously from 2004 (Table 5). Because EGIST locates in the pelvic cavity, particularly adjacent to the female genital tract, the patient's chief complaints may be compression to local organs leading to symptoms such as urinary frequency and constipation, or a mass with no symptoms. This coincides with the case we presented, in wich the main symptom was a sensation of vaginal mass and constipation. Other alterations that appear with more frequency as a vaginal mass are the cyst (Gartner's duct cysts, Mullerian cysts, bartholin's gland cysts) or recto-vaginal septum endometriosis. The age of diagnosis, 75 years is the elderly of the cases reported. In the eleven cases published the median age was 55.

The combined vaginal and rectal examination is essential in the diagnosis of recto-vaginal masses to determine the size, mobility and consistency of the tumor. In our case we found a soft, cystic, multi-lobed and not fixed tumor, but in other reported cases, the consistency was hard, that may be related to the size and degree of malignancy.

Transvaginal ultrasound is the most widely used imaging test to complete the diagnosis. A solid mass with low eco levels, similar to the uterine fibroid, is the most characteristic ultrasonographic data. NMRI and CT scans can help to determine the origin, size and relationships of the mass and the overall assessment of the pelvis. In our case, NMRI confirmed the origin of mass in the wall of the rectum.

Histollogically, EGIST often presents as spindle cells and therefore might be excluded from the differential diagnosis of spindle-cell neoplasms and could be confused with the more common leiomyoma or leiomyosarcoma (Lam et al., 2006, Mettinen et al., 2001). Some authors reported that immunohistochemistry with antibodies against *c-kit* protein (CD 117) and CD 34 is reliable and valuable for diagnosis of EGIST (Connolly et al., 2003; De Matteo et al., 2000; Saund et al., 2004). GIST typically expresses CD117, often CD34 and sometimes SMA and S-100, but its expressions vary depending on different sites.

Since the incidence of rectal-vaginal GIST is much lower than that of GIST in the stomach or small intestine, the clinicopathological profiles have not yet been accurately characterised, and there is therefore the tendency to validate the same prognostic factors for the latter as for such tumors at other sites, particularly gastric GIST. The most important and easily applicable histological criteria for prediction of GIST are its size and mitotic rate. A rate of ≤ 5 mitoses per 50 HPF is commonly used as a limit for a tumor with expected benign behaviour, and according to a large study, this can discriminate between benign and malignant tumors, especially gastric GIST.(Miettinen, M. et al, 1999). Tumors of 2 cm in diameter are generally expected to behave in a benign fashion. Tumors of 5 cm - 10 cm in diameter have a better prognosis tan those of > 10 cm in diameter. Degrees of cellularity and atipia have also been suggested as useful criteria.

It is generally agreed that complete surgical resection with negative tumor margins is the principal curative procedure for primary and non-metastatic tumors, particularly for those at a low risk. Neoadjuvance with *imatinib mesilate (Gleevec™)* may enhance the resectability of inoperable malignant GIST and may allow for optimal surgical timing. Therapy with *imatinib* is also used in the adjuvant post-operative treatment of tumors at a high risk or in cases of incomplete surgical resection. In five of the eleven cases surgery was the treatment done as first option, in two more cases (like the one we report) tumor escision and treatment with *imatinib mesylate* was established. Only in one case, there was evidence of metastatic disease, and treatment with *imatinib mesylate* was the therapeutic choice. In ten of the eleven cases reported, the diagnosis of the tumor was before evidence of metastatic disease, probably because the location in the rectovaginal septum affords an early detection.

Author (publication year)	**Age (years)**	**Tumor size (cm)**	**Treatment**	**Mitosis (/50 HPF)**	***Kit* (CD117)**	**CD34**	**Outcome**
Nasu (2004)	54	8.5	Surgery	5-10	+	+	Alive and well 13 months
Ceballos (2004)	75	4.5	Surgery	12-15	+	+	Recurrence 7.5 years
Weppler (2005)	66	8	*Imatinib*	>5	+	+	Not described
Takano (2006)	38	7	Surgery	1-2	+	+	Alive and well 12 months
Lam (2006)	36	4	Not described	15	+	+	Recurrence 2 years
Lam (2006)	48	6	Not described	12	+	+	Recurrence 10 years
Lam (2006)	61	8	Not described	16	+	+	Not described
Nagase (2007)	42	3.5	Surgery	<1	+	+	Alive and well 4 years
Nagase (2007)	66	5	Surgery+*Imatinib*	2-3	+	+	Alive and well 6 months
Zang (2009)	42	8	Surgery	10	+	+	Alive and well 6 months
Marcos (2010), the current case	75	5	Surgery+*Imatinib*	16	+	+	Alive and well till now

Table 5. Clinicopathologic features of eleven reported cases of EGISTs presenting as a vaginal mass (Zang, 2009).

As lymph nodes metastasis occurs infrequently (<10%), extensive lymphadenectomy need not to be done (Miettinen, M. et al, 1999). But despite complete resection with pathologically confirmed negative margins, the majority of tumors recur. In the eleven published cases, five recurred from several months to ten years after primitive treatment. While the majority of patients initially benefit from tyrosine kinase inhibitors, it is now clear that resistance commonly develops. Indeed, the median time to progression on *imatinib mesylate* is 2 years (De Matteo et al., 2007).

In our case, the final histological study revealed a gastrointestinal stromal tumor of high risk of malignancy (16 mitotic figures per 50 high power fields). We used *Gleevec™* as neoadjuvant therapy. The patient showed good tolerance to the drug. Evolution has been very favorable, almost three years have passed and our patient is alive and free of disease.
The lack of a large series of patients under long-term follow-up observations makes it difficult to assess the necessary extent of surgical resection and the indication for treatment with *imatinib*.

3. Conclusion

In the past years there have been significant developments in the understanding of GISTs and their response to therapy. Many questions remain unanswered and new issues have arisen as the benefits of *imatinib mesylate* therapy are revealed.
EGISTs that present as gynecologic masses are rare but may be more common than is currently recognized. Misdiagnosis may lead to an inappropriate therapy because conventional radiotherapy and chemotherapy are not effective in the treatment of GISTs, whereas *imatinib mesylate (Gleevec™)* has a proven role in managing these tumors. Thus, it is important and necessary to consider EGISTs in the differential diagnosis of mesenchymal neoplasms in the vulvovaginal-rectovaginal septum. The most common symptom is due to compression of adjacent organs, discomfort, feeling of lump, dyspareunia or constipation The differential diagnosis is done with leiomyomas and vaginal cysts (Gartner's duct cysts, Mullerian cysts, bartholin's gland cysts). GIST typically expresses CD117, often CD34 and sometimes SMA and S-100, leading to the definitive diagnosis in the biopsy samples. The prognosis is determined by the size and mitotic count. Treatment relies on surgical excision of the tumor, and *imatinib mesylate* has shown efficacy as neoadjuvant and adjuvant monotherapy.

4. Acknowledgment

We want to thank the Surgery and Pathology Department of our hospital for their help in the management of this case.

5. References

Ceballos, K.M. ; Francis, J.A. & Mazurka, J.L. (2004). Gastrointestinal stromal tumor presenting as a recurrent vaginal mass. *Archives of Patholgy and Laboratory Medicine,* Vol.128, No.12 (December 2004), pp.1442-1444, ISSN 0003-9985.

Connolly, E. M. ; Gaffney, E. & Reynolds, J. V. (2003). Gastrointestinal stromal tumors. British *Journal of Surgery,* Vol.90, No.10, (October 2003), pp.1178-1186, ISSN 1365-2168.

De Matteo, R. ; Lewis, J. ; Leung, D. ; Mudan, S. ; Woodruff, & J. Brennan, M. (2000). Two hundred gastrointestinal stroma tumours. Recurrence patterns and prognostic factors of survival. *Annals of Surgery,* Vol.231, No.1, (January 2000), pp. 51-58, ISSN 0003-4932.

De Matteo, R. ; Marki, R. ; Singer, S. ; Gonen, M. ; Brennan, M. & Antonescu, C. (2007). Results of tyrosine kinase inhibitor therapy followed by surgical resection for metastatic gastrointestinal stromal tumour. *Annals of Surgery,* Vol.245, No.3, (March 2007), pp. 347-352, ISSN 0003-4932.

Fletcher, C.D. ; Berman, J.J. ; Corless, C. ; Gorstein, F. ; Lasota, J. ; Longley, B.J. et al. (2002). Diagnosis of gastrointestinal stromal tumors : a consensus approach. *Human Pathology,* Vol.33, No.5, (May 2002), pp. 459-465, ISSN 0046-8177.

Hellan, M. & Maker, V. (2006). Transvaginal excision of a large rectal stromal tumour: an alternative. *Americal Journal of Surgery,* Vol.191, No.1, (January 2006), pp.121-123, ISSN 0002-9610.

Lam, M.; Corless, C.; Goldblum, J.; Heinrich, M.; Downs-Kelly, E. & Rubin, B. (2006) Extragastrointestinal stromal tumours presenting as vulvovaginal/rectovaginal septal masses: A diagnostic pitfall. *International Journal of Gynecological Pathology,* Vol.25, No.3, (July 2006), pp. 288-292, ISSN 0277-1691.

Marcos, J.; Román, M.J.; Esteve, N.; Saco, A.; Piñero, O.; Candela, A.; López, J.A.; Muci, T. & Martínez, J.C. (2010). Gastrointestinal stromal tumor of the rectovaginal septum: a diagnostic challenge. *Progresos de Obstetricia y Ginecología,* Vol.53, No.7, (July 2010), pp. 288-291, ISSN 0304-5013.

Miettinen, M.; Monihan, J.M.; Sarlomo-Rikala, M.; Kovatich, A.J.; Carr, N.J.; Emory, T.S.; et al. (1999). Gastrointestinal stromal tumors/smooth muscle tumors (GISTs) primary in the omentum and mesentery: clinicopathologic and immunohistochemical study of 26 cases. *The American Journal of Surgical Pathology,* Vol.9, No.23, (September 1999), pp.1109-1118, ISSN 0147-5185.

Miettinen, M:, Furlong, M.; Sarlomo-Rikala, M.; Burke, A.; Sobin, L.H. & Lasota, J.(2001). Gastrointestinal stromal tumors, intramural leiomyomas, and leiomyosarcomas in the rectum and anus: a clinicopathologic, immunohistochemical, and molecular genetic study of 144 cases. *The American Journal of Surgical Pathology,* Vol.25, No.9, (September, 2001), pp. 1121-1133, ISSN 0147-5185.

Mussi, C.; Jakob, J.; Wardelmann, E.; Reichardt, P.; Casali P.G. & Fiore, M. (2008). Gastrointestinal stromal tumor of the rectum and rectovaginal space: A retrospective review [abstract 10560]. *Journal of Clinical Oncology,* Vol.26, No.2, (May 2008), pp. 347-352, ISSN 1527-7755.

Nagase, S.; Mikami, Y.; Moriya, T.; Niikura, H.; Yoshinaga, K.; Takano, T. et al. (2007). Vaginal stromal tumors with histologic and immunohistochemical feature of gastrointestinal stromal tumor: two cases and review of the literature. *International Journal of Gynecological Cancer.* Vol.17, No.4, (July-August 2007),pp.928-933, ISSN 1048-891X.

Nickl, N. (2004). Gastrointestinal stromal tumors: new progress, new questions. *Current Opinion in Gastroenterology,* Vol.20, No.5, (September 2004), pp. 482-487, ISSN 0267-1379.

Nasu, K.; Ueda, T.; Kai, S.; Anai, H.; Kimura, Y.; Yokoyama, S. et al. (2004). Gastrointstinal stromal tumor arising in the rectovaginal septum. *International Journal of Gynecological Cancer,* Vol.14, No.3, (March 2004), pp.373-377, ISSN 1048-891X.

Parck, C.K.; Lee, E.J.; Kim, M.; Lim, H.; Choi, D.; Noh, J.H. et al. (2008). Prognostic stratification og high-risk gasrrointestinal stromal tumours in the era of targeted therapy. *Annals of Surgery,* Vol.247, No.6, (June 2008), pp.1011-1018, ISSN 0003-4932.

Pasku, D. ; Karantanas, A. ; Giannikaki, E. ; Tzardi, M. ; Velivassakis, E. & Katonis, P. (2008). Bilateral gluteal metastatses from a misdiagnosed intrapelvic gastroinestinal stromal tumor. *World Journal of Surgical Oncology*. Vol.139, No.6, (December 2008), ISSN 14777819.

Pidhorecky, I. ; Cheneky, R.T. ; Kraybill, W.G. & Gibbs, J.F. (2000). Gastrointestinal stromal tumors : current diagnosis, biologic behaviour, and management. *Annals of Surgical Oncology*, Vol.7, No.9, (September 2000), pp.705-712. ISSN 1068-9265.

Raut, C. ; Morgan, J. ; Ashley, S. (2007). Current issues in gastrointestinal stromal tumors: incidence, molecular biology, and contemporary treatment of localized and advanced disease. *Current opinion in Gastroenterology*, Vol.2, No.23, (March 2007), pp.149-158, ISSN 0267-1379.

Reid, R.; Bulusu, R.; Buckels, J.; Carroll, N.; Eatock, M.; Geh, I. et al. (2005). Guidelines for the management of gastrointestinal stromal tumours (GISTs). Available from: http://www.augis.org/news/articles/gist mngmnt gdlns 071205 final.pdf.

Ronellenfitsch, U.; Mussi, C.; Wardelmann, E.; Jakob, J.; Fumagalli, E.; Tamborini, E. et al. (2008). Surgery in patients with metastatic or recurrent gastrointestinal stromal tumours (GIST) upon best response o limited progression following imatinib therapy [abstract 10555]. *Journal of Clinical Oncology*, Vol.26, Supplement, (May 2008), ISSN 1527-7755.

Saund, M.; Demetri, G. & Ashley, S. (2004). Gastrointestinal stromal tumours. Small intestine. *Current Opinion in Gastroenterology*, Vol.20, No.2, (March 2004), pp.89-94, ISSN 0267-1379.

Taniguchi, M.; Nishida, T.; Hirota, S.; Isozaki, K.; Ito, T.; Nomur, T. et al. (1999). Effect of c-kit mutation on prognosis of gastrintestinal stromal tumors. *Cancer Research*, Vol.59, No.9, (September 1999), pp.4297-4300, ISSN 0008-5472.

Takano, M.; Saito, K.; Kita, T.; Furuya, K.; Aida, S. & Kikuchi, Y. (2006). Preoperative needle biopsy and immunohistochemical analysis for gastrointestinal stromal tumor of the rectum mimicking vaginal leiomyoma. *International Journal of Gynecological Cancer*, Vol.16, No.2, (March-April 2006), pp.927-930, ISSN 1048-891X.

Tooru, O.; Jum, K.; Takahiro, S.; Mikio, F.; Shiro, N.; Tetsuhiko, M. et al. (2001). A case of gastrointestinal stromal tumour of the rectovaginal septum. *Journal of Japan Surgical Association*, Vol.62, No.4, (April 2001), pp.988-991, ISSN1345-2843.

Valera, Z.; Sánchez, M.; Díaz, C.; Blanco, M.A.; Socas, M. & Serrano, I. (2008). GIST rectal. *Revista Española de Enfermedades Digestivas*, Vol.100, No.6, (June 2008), pp.374-375, ISSN 1130-0108.

Verma, J.; Younus, D.; Styr-Norman, A.E.; Haynes, M.; Blackstein, D. & the Sarcoma Disease Site Group. (2006). Imatinib Mesylate (Gleevec™) for the treatment of adult patients with unresecable or metastatic gastrointestinal stromal tumours: A clinical practice guideline. Evidence-based series. A Quality initiative of the Program in Evidence-Based Care, Cancer Care Ontario (April 2006). Section 1:1-3.

Verweij, J.; Casali, P.G.; Zalcberg, J.; LeCesbe, A.; Reichardt, P.; Blay, J.Y., et al. (2004). Progression-free survival in gastrointestinal stromal tumours with high dose imatinib: randomised trial. *The Lancet*, Vol.364, No.9440, (september 2004), pp. 1127-1134, ISSN 0140-6736.

Weppler, E.H. & Gaertner, E.M.(2005). Malignant extragastrointestinal stromal tumor presenting as a vaginal mass: report of an unusual case with a literature review.

International Journal of Gynecological Cancer. Vol.15, No.6, (November 2005), pp.1169-1172, ISSN 1048-891X.

Yamamoto, H.; Oda, Y.; Kawaguchi, K.; Nakamura, N.; Takahira, T.; Tamiya, S. et al. (2004). C-kit and PDGFRA mutations in extragastrointestinal stromal tumor (gastrointestinal stromal tumor of the soft tissue). *The American Journal of Surgical Pathology,* Vol.28, No.4, (April, 2004), pp. 479-488, ISSN 0147-5185.

Zalupski, M.; Metch, B.; Balcerzak, S.; Fletcher, W.S.; Chapman, R.; Bonnet, J.D. et al. (1991). Phase III comparison of doxorubicin and dacarbazine given by bolus versus infusion in patients with soft-tissue sarcomas: a Southwest Oncology Group study. *Journal of the National Cancer Institute,* Vol.83, No.13, (July 1991), pp. 926-932, ISSN 0027-8874.

Zang, W.; Peng, Z. & Xu, L. (2009). Extragastrointestinal stromal tumor arising in the rectovaginal septum: Report og an unusual case with literature review. *Gynecologic Oncology,* Vol.113, No.3, (June 2009), pp.399-401, ISSN 0090-8258.

The Significance of the Ki-67 Labeling Index, the Expression of c-kit, p53, and bcl-2, and the Apoptotic Count on the Prognosis of Gastrointestinal Stromal Tumor

Keishiro Aoyagi, Kikuo Kouhuji and Kazuo Shirouzu
Department of Surgery, Kurume University School of Medicine
Japan

1. Introduction

Gastrointestinal stromal tumor (GIST) express the cell surface transmembrane receptor KIT that has tyrosine kinase activity and is the protein product of the KIT proto-oncogene c-kit. Activation or gain-infunction mutation in the *c-kit* gene has been identified in the majority of GIST cases.

The mutation results in the constitutive activation of KIT signaling, which leads to uncontrolled cell proliferation and resistance to apoptosis. Somatic mutation in the *c-kit* gene of GIST has been reported to be associated with aggressive progression and poor prognosis. The diameter of the tumor and the mitotic index have been reported as useful indices of the biological malignancy of GISTs. However, a few cases in the benign group had high cellularity, ulcer formation or metastasis/recurrence. Therefore, other indices of the biological malignancy of GISTs are thought to be needed.

Recently, the Ki-67 labeling index, p53 immunoreaction, and bcl-2 overexpression have each been reported to be useful in predicting the potential malignancy in GISTs. In this chapter, the reliabilities of the Ki-67 labeling index, the expression of c-kit, p53, and bcl-2, and the apoptotic count for predicting potential malignancy were assessed.

2. Patients and methods

2.1 Patients

Twelve patients with gastric or small intestine stromal tumors who underwent surgical resection at our department; 11 involving the stomach and the other one involving the small intestine, were retrospective analyzed. Nine patients were male, and three were female (age range, 47-79 years; mean age, 62.8±10.5 years). The series consisted of seven patients with GIST in the upper body of the stomach, one in the upper body of the remnant stomach, two in the middle body of the stomach, one in the antrum, and one in the jejunum. Four patients who either had metastasis at the time of the initial operation or recurrence after operation were classified as the metastasis/recurrence group, whereas the other eight patients are surviving without postoperative recurrence.

2.2 Clinicopathological study

As prognostic determinants, we examined mean tumor diameter, and the mitotic index (the frequency of mitosis in 50 visual fields at a magnification of ×400). We used Amin's classification of malignant (mitotic index >5/50 high power fields (HPF), irrespective of tumor diameter), borderline (mitotic index <5/50 HPF and tumor diameter >5 cm), and benign (mitotic index <5/50 HPF and tumor diameter <5 cm).

2.3 Immunohistochemical staining

After an initial review of all available hematoxylin and eosin (H&E)-stained slides of the surgical specimen, we selected paraffin blocks in which the central region of the tumor was clearly revealed, from each case, to study. Serial 4-μm-thick sections were recut from each block. One section from each block was stained with H&E. Other sections were immunostained for c-kit, CD34, vimentin, α-smooth muscle stain (SMA), desmin, S-100, Ki-67, p53, and bcl-2. Immunostaining was performed using the dextran polymer method for c-kit, CD34, α-SMA, desmin, and S-100. Anti-human c-kit rabbit polyclonal antibody (DAKO, Kyoto, Japan), anti-human CD34 mouse monoclonal antibody (DAKO), anti-human vimentin mouse monoclonal antibody (DAKO), anti-human α-SMA mouse monoclonal antibody (DAKO), anti-human desmin mouse monoclonal antibody (DAKO), or anti-human S-100 rabbit polyclonal antibody (DAKO) was used as the primary antibody. The deparaffinized sections were irradiated by microwaves for 15 min (400W; H2800 microwave processor, Energy Beam Sciences) at 90℃ and were incubated with 0.03% H_2O_2 / methanol for 30 minutes for blocking endogenous peroxidase activity. After washing in phosphate buffered saline (PBS), the sections were incubated with the primary antibody for 30 minutes at room temperature. After rewashing, the sections were further incubated with peroxidase-labeled dextran conjugated anti-mouse and anti-rabbit immunoglobulin goat polyclonal antibody (DAKO) for 30 min at room temperature. After washing again , the sections were developed with chromogen 3,3′- diaminobenzidine tetrahydrochloride.

Immunostaining was performed using the avidin-biotin complex method for Ki-67, p53, and bcl-2. Anti-human Ki-67 mouse monoclonal antibody (MM1 Novocastra, Newcastle, UK), anti-human p53 mouse monoclonal antibody (Do-7 Novocastra), or anti-human bcl-2 mouse monoclonal antibody (Novocastra) was used as the primary antibody. The deparaffinized sections were heated in an autoclave at 120℃ for 5 minutes in citric acid buffer (2 mmol/l citric acid and 9 mmol/l trisodium citrate dehydrate, pH6.0) and incubated with 0.03% H_2O_2 / methanol for 30 minutes for blocking endogenous peroxidase activity. After washing in PBS, nonspecific binding was blocked by incubating the sections with normal animal serum for 20 minutes. The sections were incubated with the primary antibody overnight at 4℃. After washing, the sections were further incubated with biotinylated second antibody for 30 minutes at room temperature. The primary antibody was detected using the avidin-biotin peroxidase complex (Vector Laboratories, Burlingame, CA) and 3-amino-9-ethylcarbazole as the chromogen. These thin sections were also counterstained with hematoxylin and mounted. For immunoreactivity of p53 and bcl-2 proteins, tissue sections with >10% immunopositive cells in 1000 tumor cells from three arbitrary microscopic fields were defined as being positive (+), and those with <10% immunoreactive tumor cells were defined as being negative (-).

The Ki-67 Index was defined as the percentage of tumor cells displaying immunoreactivity in 1000 cells in a ×100 magnified field from five arbitrary microscopic fields.

2.4 TUNEL staining

Apoptotic tumor cells were detected by using the terminal deoxynucleotide transferase-mediated deoxyuridine triphosphate biotin nick-end labeling (TUNEL) method. The Apo Tag *in situ* detection kit (Intergen, Purchase, NY) was used according to the manufacturer's instructions. The apoptotic count was defined as the mean number of TUNEL-positive cells in a ×400 magnified field from 10 arbitrary microscopic fields.

2.5 Statistical analysis

Student's t -test and the chi-square test were used to analyze the data for significant differences, and differences were considered statistically significant when $P < 0.05$. Continuous variables were presented as the mean ± SD.

3. Clinicopathological study

3.1 Clinicopathological features

In six cases, the lesion was incidentally discovered during a routine screening examination. The other six cases were symptomatic and presented epigastric pain, abdominal discomfort, anemia, vomiting, an abnormal shadow on chest X-ray, or tumor palpable, respectively. The lesion size ranged from 18 to 200 mm in diameter (mean size 55.0±44.5 mm) . The GIST in the jejunum was palpable. The macroscopic aspects of GIST in the jejunum are a smooth surface, gray color, pseudocapsule, and exophitic growth. We found one case with liver metastasis, one with lung metastasis, one with bone metastasis, and no cases with lymph node metastasis at the time of surgery (Table 1).

3.2 Histology and malignancy

A Mitotic Index of > 5/50 HPF was seen in five cases and <5/50HPF in the other seven cases. A high cellularity was seen in four cases, a middle cellularity in four cases, and a low cellularity was seen in the other four cases. Concerning the degree of anaplasia, a high degree was seen in three cases, a middle degree in four cases, and a low degree was seen in the other five cases. The number of cases with ulcer formation, cases with necrosis, cases with bleeding in the tumor, and the number of cases with mucosal invasion by tumor cells was four, one, four, and one, respectively. The numbers in the malignant group, borderline group, and in the benign group were five, two, and five, respectively. Three of four cases in the metastasis/recurrence group were malignant group, but other one was benign group. All four cases in the metastasis/recurrence group had ulcer formation and high cellularity. One case with necrosis and mucosal invasion had lung metastasis. Two of four cases with bleeding in the tumor was in the metastasis/recurrence group. Two of three cases with high atypia was in the metastasis/recurrence group. In the malignant group, the tumor size was >5 cm in diameter in three cases, the cellularity in four cases was middle or high, three cases had ulcer formation, three cases had bleeding in the tumor, and one case had necrosis in the tumor with mucosal invasion by tumor cells. In the boderline group, the cellularity was middle or low, the degree of anaplasia was high or low, one case had bleeding in the tumor, and there was no ulcer formation, no necrosis in the tumor, and no mucosal invasion. In the benign group, the tumor size was 3 cm or less in diameter. The cellularity was low in two cases, middle in two cases, and high in one case. The degree of anaplasia was low in three cases, middle in two cases, and high in no case. One case with bone metastasis had ulcer formation . There was no necrosis, no bleeding in the tumor, and no mucosal invasion (Table 1).

Case	Site	Mitosis(HPF)	Size(mm)	Cellularity	Ulcer	Necrosis	Bleeding	Atypia	Invasion	*Metastasis	Malignancy
1	U	10/10	80x60	High	+	-	-	High	-	Liver	Malignant
2	U	6/50	40x33	Middle	-	-	+	Low	-	None	Malignant
3	M	6/50	18x12	Low	-	-	-	Middle	-	None	Malignant
4	U**	13/10	120x100	High	+	+	+	High	+	Left lung	Malignant
5	U	-	52x48	Middle	-	-	+	High	-	None	Borderline
6	U	4/50	60x45	Low	-	-	-	Low	-	None	Borderline
7	U	-	30x30	Low	-	-	-	Low	-	None	Benign
8	L	-	30x30	Middle	-	-	-	Middle	-	None	Benign
9	U	3/50	25x25	High	+	-	-	Middle	-	bone	Benign
10	M	-	25x20	Low	-	-	-	Low	-	None	Benign
11	U	3/50	20x20	Middle	-	-	-	Low	-	None	Benign
12	J	10/10	200x160x120	High	+	-	+	Middle	-	None	Malignant

U: upper body of the stomach, M: middle body of the stomach, L: lower body of the stomach, J: jejunum, *mucosal invasion, **upper part of the remnant stomach

Table 1. Histological findings and malignancy

The diameter of the tumor and the mitotic index have been reported as useful indices of biological malignancy in GISTs. We used Amin's classification, preparing evaluation criteria based on the pattern of mitosis and the diameter of the tumor. Mucosal invasion, bleeding, necrosis, and high degree of anaplasia were not recognized in the benign group. However, one case with bone metastasis in benign group had high cellularity and ulcer formation. Therefore, the diameter of the tumor and the mitotic index were not only useful indices of biological malignancy, but also cellularity, ulcer formation, necrosis, bleeding in the tumor, anaplasia, and mucosal invasion.

3.3 Treatment

Concerning the treatment, local resection was performed in eight cases, and in five of these cases, laparoscopic local resection was performed. In the other four cases, proximal gastrectomy with intrahepatic arterial infusion of adriamycin, resection of the remnant stomach with left lower lobectomy of the lung, local resection with radiation for bone metastasis and partial resection of the jejunum including the tumor were performed (Table 2).

3.4 Prognosis

Concerning survival, one patient with lung metastasis received resection of the remnant stomach with left lower lobectomy of the lung, and later died of intra-abdominal and right lung recurrence at 35 months later. One patient with multiple liver metastasis received proximal gastrectomy with intrahepatic arterial infusion of adriamycin, recurrence in the abdomen was recognized, removed and imatinib was administered from 41 months, but died of peritoneal metastasis at 58 months after the first surgery. The prognosis of the patient with bone metastasis received local resection with radiation was unknown. The patient with the large GIST in the jejunum received partial resection of the jejunum including the tumor, recurrence in the liver was recognized and imatinib was administered from 25 months, local recurrence was recognized in the small intestine and removed at 45 months, and was still alive at 75 months after the first surgery (Table 2). The other patients are still alive and disease-free.

Case	Age	Sex	Treatment	Recurrence	Imatinib	Prognosis
1	49	M	Proximal gastrectomy Intrahepatic arterial infusion*	41M peritoneum	+	58M dead
2	68	M	Laparoscopic local resection	-	-	8M alive
3	63	M	Laparoscopic local resection	-	-	120M alive
4	55	M	Resection of the remnant stomach Lt. lower lobectomy of the lung	30M peritoneum,lung	-	35M dead
5	64	M	Laparoscopic local resection	-	-	79M alive
6	66	F	Local resection	-	-	8M alive
7	70	F	Laparoscopic local resection	-	-	8M alive
8	47	M	Local resection	-	-	128M alive
9	78	F	Local resection, Radiation	-	-	- -
10	51	M	Laparoscopic local resection	-	-	49M alive
11	63	M	Local resection	-	-	34M alive
12	79	M	Partial resection of jejunum Tumor resection	25M Liver, 45M Local recurrence	+	75M alive

*: Intrahepatic arterial infusion of adriamycin

Table 2. Treatment and prognosis

4. Immunohistochemical staining

4.1 c-kit expression

All patients were positive for vimentin expression. Seven patients were positive for c-kit expression. Nine patients were positive for CD34 expression. In the seven c-kit-positive cases, six patients were also positive for CD34 expression. Two patients were positive for α-SMA expression. All patients were negative for both desmin and S-100 expression. All four cases in the metastasis/recurrence group were positive for c-kit expression (Table 3). The positive rate of c-kit in the malignant group was 100% (five of five), in the borderline group, it was 50% (one of two), and in the benign group, it was 20% (one of five; Table 4)).The positive rate of c-kit in the malignant group was significantly higher than in the borderline and benign group ($P < 0.05$). Mean tumor size in the c-kit -positive group was 76.4 ± 62.2 mm and c-kit-negative group was 33.0 ± 21.0 mm (Table 5).The mean tumor diameter in the c-kit-positive group was higher than that in the c-kit-negative group.

Concerning any correlation between cellularity and c-kit expression, the positive rate of c-kit in the high group was 100% (four of four), in the middle group was 50% (two of four), and in the low group was 25% (one of four). Concerning any correlation between the degree of anaplasia and the c-kit expression, the positive rate of c-kit in the high group was 100%

(three of three), in the middle group was 75% (three of four), and in the low group was 20% (one of five). The positive rate of c-kit in cases with ulcer formation was 100% (four of four), and in cases without ulcer formation it was 37.5% (three of eight). The positive rate of c-kit in cases with bleeding in the tumor was 100% (four of four), and in cases without bleeding in the tumor, it was 37.5% (three of eight). All malignant cases, cases with high cellularity, cases with high degree of anaplasia, cases with ulcer formation, and cases with bleeding in the tumor were positive for c-kit expression.

Immunohistochemistry analyses have been reported to show a positivity reaction to CD34 in > 80% of cases, and to the c-kit in 95-100%. In our study, the positive rate to CD34 was 83.3%, and to the c-kit it was 66.7%. Therefore, the positive rate to the c-kit was lower than in other reports. However, all other reported cases lacked immunohistochemical evidence of smooth muscle or neural differentiation. Hirota reported that some GISTs lacked immunoreactivity to c-kit without immunohistochemical evidence of smooth muscle or neural differentiation. Many GISTs showed a positivity to CD34 recognized in endothelial cells and in interstitial cells of Cajal. The positive rate to α-SMA was 16.7% in our cases. Hirota reported that from 20 to 30% of GISTs were positive to α-SMA. Somatic mutation in the c-kit gene of GIST has been reported to be associated with aggressive progression and poor prognosis. Ernst reported that the 3-year survival rate of cases without mutation in c-kit was >65%, but that of cases with mutation in c-kit it was < 30%. In our cases, all malignant cases were c-kit positive, and in the benign group only one case which had bone metastais was c-kit positive. The average diameter in the c-kit-positive group was higher than that in the c-kit-negative group.

The expression of c-kit was considered to reflect the malignancy of the GIST. It has recently been clarified that the autoactivation of tyrosin kinase caused by upregulation of the c-kit gene was related essentially to proliferation in the GIST cells, and imatinib, which inhibits the autoactivation of tyrosine kinase, has been reported to be effective as a molecule-targeting treatment. Although adjuvant use of imatinib is currently under evaluation, it is expected to be a useful treatment for an unresectable GIST or for a patient with metastasis/recurrence.

4.2 The Ki-67 labelling index

Immunoreactivity to Ki-67 was seen in the nucleus of tumor cells (Fig. 1). The Ki-67 labeling index ranged between 4.7 to 49.8 (mean 25.4±15.9; Table 3). In the metastasis/recurrence group, the Ki-67 labeling index in patient with liver metastasis was 49.8, in patient with bone metastasis was 26.8, in patient with lung metastasis, it was 40.2, and in small intestinal GIST patient with recurrence in the liver, it was 34.6. The Ki-67 labeling index in the malignant group was 35.3±11.0, in the borderline group 37.5±9.40, and in the benign group was 10.6±9.26 (Table 4). The Ki-67 labeling index in the malignant group was significantly higher than that in the benign group ($p < 0.01$). The Ki-67 labeling index in the c-kit-positive cases was 35.3±10.2 and in c-kit- negative cases was 11.4±11.0. The Ki-67 labeling index in the c-kit positive cases was significantly higher than that in the c-kit-negative cases ($p < 0.01$).

The Ki-67 labeling index in the c-kit-positive cases was 35.3±10.2 and in c-kit- negative cases was 11.4±11.0 (Table 5). The Ki-67 labeling index in the c-kit positive cases was significantly higher than that in the c-kit-negative cases ($p < 0.01$).

AgNOR staining, DNA ploidy pattern of the nucleus, bromodeoxyuridine labeling index, Ki-67 labeling index, proliferative cell nuclear antigen (PCNA), and p53 staining have each been reported to be a useful marker as an index of malignancy in GIST. Especially, the Ki-67 labeling index has recently been used as an excellent index of cell growth. The mitotic index reflects the M stage of mitosis only; however, because the Ki-67 labeling index can recognize most proliferating cells in stages G1, S, and G2, it is considered to be more appropriate as an objective index of the malignancy in GIST. Shimoda et al. reported that the Ki-67 labeling index was > 10% in all patients with a mitotic index > 10/200 HPF. Wang et al. reported that the prognosis of GIST was significantly poor when the Ki-67 labeling index was 10% or more. Nagasako et al reported that the maximum tumor diameter, mitotic index, and Ki-67 labeling index were useful as indices of malignancy for a gastric stromal tumor. In the present study, all four cases of the metastasis/recurrence group showed a high Ki-67 labeling index (49.8, 26.8, 40.2 and 34.6), and the mean Ki-67 labeling index in the malignant group was higher than that in the benign group. Even in the benign group, one case with bone metastasis showed a high Ki-67 labeling index (26.8), and this case showed high cellularity and had ulcer formation. Such a case should be carefully followed postoperatively. The mean Ki-67 labeling index in the c-kit-positive cases was higher than that in the c-kit-negative cases. The Ki-67 labeling index was considered to be a useful marker of malignancy in GIST.

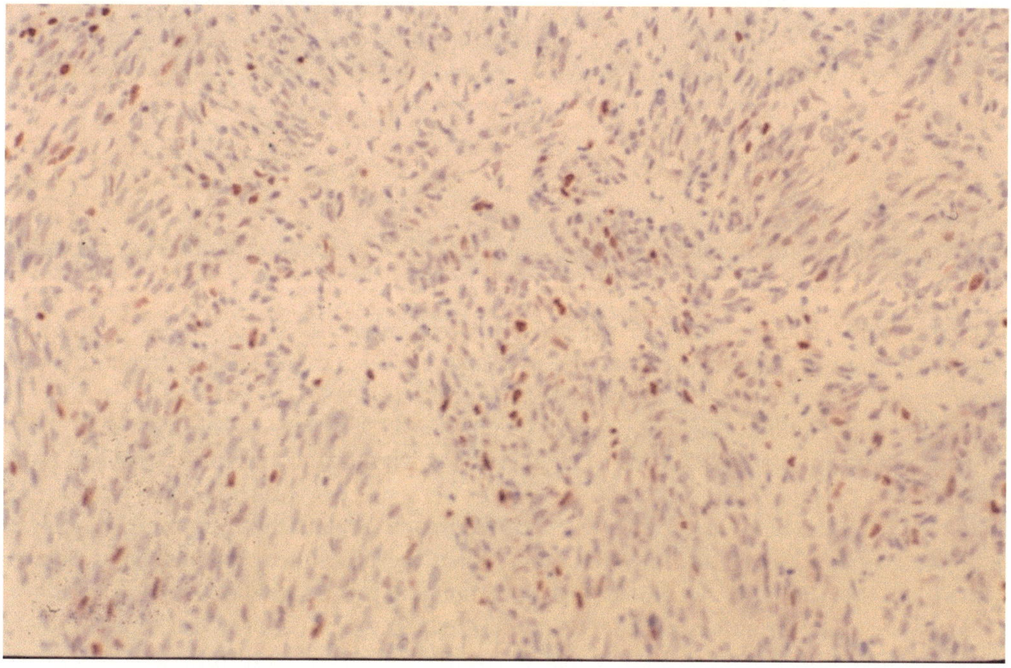

Fig. 1. Immunoreactivity for Ki-67; Immunostaining for Ki-67 was confined to almost the entire nucleus (×200)

4.3 p53 expression

The immunoreactivity of p53 was also mainly identified in the nucleus (Fig. 2). Four patients were positive for p53 expression. Three cases of the metastasis/recurrence group were positive for p53 expression. The positive rate of p53 in the malignant group was 60.0% (three of five), in the borderline group was 50.0% (one of two), and in the benign group was 0%(zero of five; Table 4). The mean tumor size in the p53-positive group was 115.0±61.9 mm and in the p53-negative group was 26.3±11.9 mm. The mean tumor size in the p53-positive group was higher than that of p53- negative group.

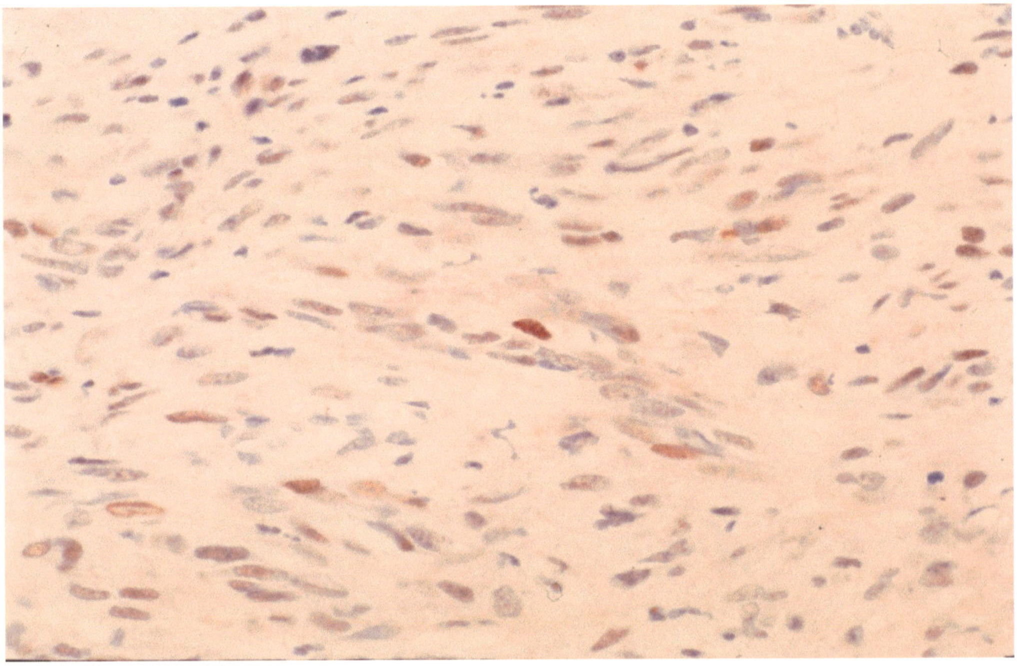

Fig. 2. p53 staining; Immunohistochemical staining with a monoclonal antibody against p53. Nuclear staining was observed in the tumor cells (×400).

The mean Ki-67 labeling index in the p53-positive group was 38.9±8.26 and in the p53-negative group was 18.6±14.6. The mean Ki-67 labeling index in the p53-positive group was significantly higher than that in the p53-negative group ($p < 0.05$).

The p53- positive rate in the c-kit-positive group was 42.9% (three of seven), and in the c-kit-negative group was 20.0% (one of five), with no significant difference between them (Table 5).

Following DNA damage, p53 protein levels rise dramatically, and the entry into S is delayed until the genomic lesions are fully repaired. When the p53 function is lost, cells enter S without appropriate DNA repair, leading to fixation and propagation of genetic alterations. p53 overexpression promotes the transcription of p21, the product of which causes growth arrest through inhibition in Cdks, which are required for G1 to S transition. p21 is induced by DNA-damaging agents that trigger G1 arrest or apoptosis in cells with wild type p53 but not in tumor cells harboring a deletion or mutation in the p53 gene. Nikaido et al. reported that survival in gastric leiomyosarcoma of p53-positive cases was significantly shorter than that of p53- negative cases, that immunohistochemical p53 positivity was correlated with malignant behavior, and that p53 immunoreaction was a prognostic variable. In our cases, three cases of the metastasis/recurrence group were positive for p53 expression. The Ki-67 labeling index in all p53 -positive cases was >30%. There was no p53-positive case in the benign group. The mean tumor diameter of the p53-positive cases was higher than that of the p53-negative cases. The mean Ki-67 labeling index of the p53-positive cases was higher than that of the p53-negative cases. The expression to p53 was considered to be a useful marker as an index of malignancy and prognosis in GIST.

4.4 bcl-2 expression

The immunoreactivity of bcl-2 was mainly identified in the cytoplasm of tumor cells (Fig. 3). Seven patients were positive for bcl-2 expression (Table 3).

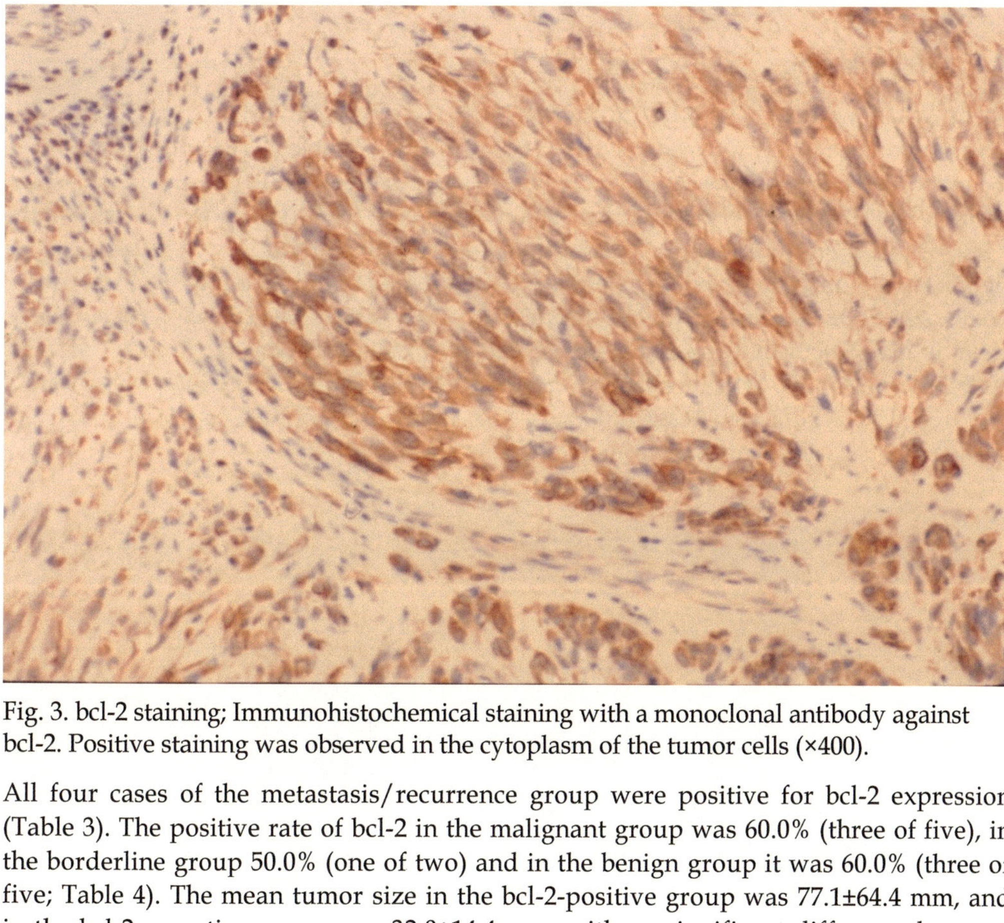

Fig. 3. bcl-2 staining; Immunohistochemical staining with a monoclonal antibody against bcl-2. Positive staining was observed in the cytoplasm of the tumor cells (×400).

All four cases of the metastasis/recurrence group were positive for bcl-2 expression (Table 3). The positive rate of bcl-2 in the malignant group was 60.0% (three of five), in the borderline group 50.0% (one of two) and in the benign group it was 60.0% (three of five; Table 4). The mean tumor size in the bcl-2-positive group was 77.1±64.4 mm, and in the bcl-2- negative group was 32.0±14.4 mm, with no significant difference between them.

The mean Ki-67 labeling index in the bcl-2-positive group was 28.3±15.8 mm, and in the bcl-2-negative group was 21.3±17.0 mm, with no significant difference between them.

The bcl-2-positive rate in the c-kit-positive group was 57.1% (four of seven), and in the c-kit-negative group was 60.0% (three of five), with no significant difference between them (Table 5).

The bcl-2-positive rate in the p53-positive group was 100% (four of four), and in the p53-negative group was 37.5% (three of eight), with no significant difference between them.

Cunningham et al. reported that the patients whose tumor demonstrated staining for bcl-2 protein had a shorter survival compared with those whose tumor did not demonstrate bcl-2. Noguchi et al. reported that overexpression in bcl-2 may play an important role in increasing the malignant potential, and furthermore, that the Ki-67 labeling index and bcl-2 overexpression may be useful in predicting malignant potential. In our study, all four cases of the metastasis/recurrence group were positive for bcl-2 expression, and all p53-positive cases were positive for bcl-2 expression. However, no significant correlation was observed between the frequency of the bcl-2 overexpression and the malignancy in the GIST, tumor diameter, or Ki-67 labeling index,

5. TUNEL staining

Positive staining was recognized in the nuclei in the apoptotic tumor cells (Fig. 4). The apoptotic count ranged between 0.1 to 3.9 (mean 1.20±1.14; Table3). The apoptotic count in the malignant group was 1.44±1.65, in the borderline group was 0.50±0.57, and in the benign group was 0.80±0.71, with no significant difference among them. The apoptotic count in the c-kit-positive group was 1.44±1.32, and in the c-kit-negative group was 0.88±0.88, with no significant difference between them (Table 5). The mean apoptotic count in the p53-positive group was 2.33±1.20, and in the p53-negative group was 0.65±0.62. The mean apoptotic count in the p53-positive group was higher than that in the p53-negative group. The mean apoptotic count in the bcl-2- positive group was 1.80±1.16, and in the bcl-2-negative group it was 0.38±0.36, with a significant difference ($p < 0.05$). All apoptotic counts of malignant group or metastasis/recurrence group were 1.0 or > 1.0.

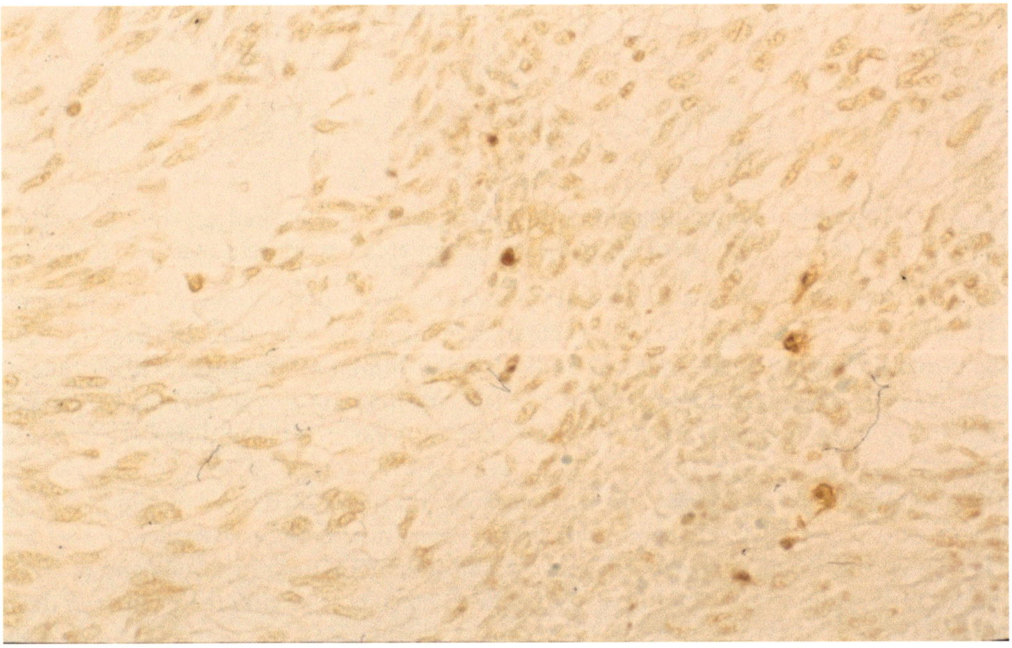

Fig. 4. TUNEL staining; TUNEL-positive staining was recognized in the nucleus of apoptotic tumor cells (×200).

Case	c-kit	CD34	Vimentin	α-SMA	Desmin	S-100	p53	bcl-2	Ki-67	Apoptosis
1	+	+	+	-	-	-	+	+	49.8	2.0
2	+	+	+	+	-	-	-	-	19.8	0.1
3	+	-	+	+	-	-	-	-	32.1	0.2
4	+	+	+	-	-	-	+	+	40.2	1.0
5	+	+	+	-	-	-	-	-	44.1	0.9
6	-	+	+	-	-	-	+	+	30.8	2.4
7	-	+	+	-	-	-	-	+	9.7	0.6
8	-	-	+	-	-	-	-	-	4.7	0.6
9	+	+	+	-	-	-	-	+	26.8	2.0
10	-	-	+	-	-	-	-	+	6.1	0.7
11	-	+	+	-	-	-	-	-	5.6	0.1
12	+	+	+	-	-	-	+	+	34.6	3.9

Table 3. Results from immunohistochemistry, Ki-67 index and the apoptotic count

	Malignant (n=5)	Borderline (n=2)	Benign (n=5)
Ki-67 Index*	35.3±11.0	37.5±9.40	10.6±9.26
Apoptotic count	1.44±1.65	0.50±0.57	0.80±0.71
p53 positive cases	3 (60.0%)	1 (50.0%)	0
bcl-2 positive cases	3 (60.0%)	1 (50.0%)	3 (60.0%)
c-kit positive cases**	5 (100%)	1 (50.0%)	1 (20.0%)

*: The Ki-67 Index in the malignant group was significantly higher than that in the benign group ($p < 0.01$).

**: The positive rate of c-kit in the malignant group was significantly higher than in the borderline and benign group ($P < 0.05$).

Table 4. Ki-67 index, Apoptotic Count and the expressions of p53, bcl-2 and c-kit according to Malignancy

Concerning apoptosis, Cunningham et al. reported that inhibition in apoptosis may be associated with malignant behavior in patients with gastrointestinal stromal/smooth muscle tumors. Yuki et al. reported that the apoptotic cell counts of leiomyosarcoma were significantly higher than those of leiomyoma, but this seems not to be a practical index for discrimination because apoptotic cell death is a rare event in gastrointestinal myogenic tumors. In our study, there was no significant difference in apoptotic count among the benign group, borderline group, and the malignant group. The mean apoptotic count in the bcl-2-positive group was higher than that in the bcl-2-negative group, and the mean apoptotic count in the p53-positive group was higher than that in the p53-negative group. p53 induces upregulation in bax protein which accelerates apoptotic death. bcl-2 protein is able to repress a number of apoptotic death programs. bax homodimerizes and forms heterodimers with bcl-2 in vivo. The ratio of bcl-2 to bax determines survival or death following an apoptotic stimulus. Therefore, if overexpressed bax countered the death repressor activity of bcl-2, and apoptosis was considered to be induced in cases that were positive for bcl-2 expression.

	c-kit-positive cases (n=7)	c-kit-negative cses (n=5)
Tumor size	76.4±62.2 mm	33.0±21.0 mm
Ki-67 Index*	35.3±10.2	11.4±11.0
Apoptotic count	1.44±1.32	0.88±0.88
p53-positive cases	3 (42.9%)	1 (20.0%)
bcl-2-positive cases	4 (57.4%)	3 (60.0%)

*: Mean Ki-67 Index in the c-kit-positive cases was significantly higher than that in the c-kit-negative cases ($p < 0.01$).

Table 5. Tumor Size, Ki-67 index, apoptotic count, and the expressions of p53 and bcl-2 according to the expression of c-kit

6. Conclusion

Here, we report the Ki-67 labeling index, the expression of c-kit, p53, bcl-2, and apoptosis in eleven gastrointestinal stromal tumors (GISTs). The positive rate of c-kit in the malignant group was higher than in the borderline and benign group . The Ki-67 labeling index in the malignant GIST group was higher than that in the benign group. The Ki-67 labeling index in the c-kit-positive group was higher than that in the c-kit-negative group. The Ki-67 labeling index in the p53-positive cases was higher than that in the p53-negative cases. The bcl-2 expression was not correlated with potential malignancy. All metastasis/recurrence cases were bcl-2 positive. The apoptotic count in the bcl-2-positive cases was higher than that in the bcl-2-negative cases. All apoptotic counts of malignant group or metastasis/recurrence group were 1.0 or > 1.0.

The high Ki-67 labeling index, the c-kit positive, the p53 over expression, the bcl-2 over expression and high apoptotic count were useful in predicting the potential malignancy of GIST.

7. References

Hirota, S. (1998). Gain-of-function mutation of c-kit in human gastrointestinal stromal tumors. *Science*, 279,577-580

Nishida T. (2000). Clinicopathological features of gastric stromal tumors. *J Exp Clin Cancer*, 19,417-425

Ernst SI. (1998). KIT mutation portends poor prognosis in gastrointestinal stromal/smooth muscle tumors. *Lab Invest*, 78,1633-1636.

Miettinen M. (2002). Evaluation of malignancy and prognosis of gastrointestinal stromal tumors. *Hum Pathol*, 33,478-483

Wang X. (2002) Gastrointestinal stromal tumors: Are they of Cajal cell origin? *Exp Mol Pathol* ,72,172-177

Hasegawa T. (2002). Gastrointestinal stromal tumors: consistent CD117 immunostaining for diagnosis and prognostic classification based on tumor size and MIB-1 grade. *Hum Pathol*, 33,669-676

Abdulkader I. ((2002). Predictors of malignant behavior in gastrointestinal stromal tumors : a clinicopathological study of 34 cases. *Eur J Surg*, 168,288-296

Shimoda T. (2002). A concept and issue of GIST (gastrointestinal stromal tumor). *Pathol Clin Med*, 20,134-140

Wang X. (2002). Helpful parameter for malignant potential of gastrointestinal stromal tumors (GIST). *Jpn J Clin Oncol*, 9,347-351

Noguchi T. (2002). Biological analysis of gastrointestinal stromal tumors. *Oncol Rep*, 9, 1277-1282

Nagasako Y. (2003). Evaluation of malignancy using Ki-67 labeling index for gastric stromal tumor. *Gastric Cancer*, 6,168-172

Cunningham RE. (2001). Apoptosis, bcl-2 expression, and p53 expression in gastrointestinal stromal/smooth muscle tumors. *Appl Immunohistochem Mol Morphol*, 9,19-23

Amin MB. (1993). Prognostic value of proliferating cell nuclear antigen index in gastric stromal tumors: correlation with mitotic count and clinical outcome. *Am J Clin Pathol*, 100,428-432

Strickland L. (2001). Gastrointestinal stromal tumors. *Cancer Control*, 8,252-261

Fujimoto Y. (2003). Clinicopathologic study of primary malignant gastrointestinal tumor of the stomach, with special reference to prognostic factors: analysis of results in 140 surgically resected patients. *Gastric Cancer*, 6, 39-48

Hirota S. (2003). Gain-of-function mutation of c-kit gene and molecular target therapy in GISTs. *Jpn J Gastroenterol*, 100,13-20

Joensuu H. (2001). Effect of the tyrosin kinase inhibitor ST1571 in a patient with a metastatic gastrointestinal tumor. *N Engl J Med*, 344,1052-1056

Nikaido T. (1995). An analysis of predicting prognostic factors of the gastric leiomyosarcoma - a comparative study of their proliferative activity using mitotic index, MIB-1, DNA flow cytometry, and p53 immunostaining. *Stomach and Intestine*, 30,1125-1132

Yuki M. (1995). Cell proliferation and cell death (apoptosis) as indices differentiating malignant from benign gastrointestinal myogenic tumors. *Jpn J Gastroenterol*, 92, 206-216

Baak JPA. (1991). Mitosis counting in tumors. *Hum Pathol*, 21,683-685

Xiong Y. (1993). p21 is a universal inhibitor of cyclin kinases. *Nature*, 366,701-704.

El-Deiry W. (1994). WAF1/CIP1 is induced in p53-mediated G1 arrest and apoptosis. *Cancer Res*, 54,1169-1174

Dulic V. (1994). p53-dependent inhibition of cyclin-dependent kinase activities in human fibroblasts during radiation-induced G1 arrest. *Cell*, 76,1013-1023

Miyashita T. (1995). Tumor suppressor p53 is a direct transcriptional activator of human bax gene. *Cell*, 80, 293-299

Boise LH. (1993). bcl-x, a bcl-2-related gene that functions as a dominant regulator of apoptotic cell death. *Cell*, 74,597-608

Oltvai ZN. (1993). Bcl-2 heterodimerizes in vivo with a conserved homolog, Bax, that accelerates programmed cell death. Cell, 27,609-619